CHILDBIRTH—WITH UNDERSTANDING

CHILDBIRTH
WITH UNDERSTANDING

A Prepared Childbirth
Program with Rooming-in

By

HERBERT THOMS, M.D.
Professor Emeritus of Obstetrics and Gynecology
Curator Yale Medical Memorabilia
Yale University

With a Foreword by
MILTON J. E. SENN, M.D.
Yale University

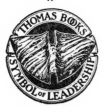

CHARLES C THOMAS • PUBLISHER
Springfield • Illinois • U.S.A.

CHARLES C THOMAS • PUBLISHER

Bannerstone House

301-327 East Lawrence Avenue, Springfield, Illinois, U.S.A.

*With THOMAS BOOKS careful attention is given to all details of
manufacturing and design. It is the Publisher's desire to present books
that are satisfactory as to their physical qualities and artistic possibilities
and appropriate for their particular use. THOMAS BOOKS will be true
to those laws of quality that assure a good name and good will.*

Printed in the United States of America

This book is dedicated to
Hazel Corbin and her associates
at the Maternity Center Association of New York

INTRODUCTION

T HIS book is concerned with those aspects of care in pregnancy and childbirth which include preparation for childbirth, rooming-in for mothers and infants, and preparation for parenthood. There are numerous papers on these and allied subjects to be found in the medical literature but nowhere in a single work is there set down the details of a comprehensive program which might be called that of "Family Centered Maternity Care" a phrase suggested by the title of Ernestine Wiedenbach's book, *Family Centered Maternity Nursing.*

It is important, also, I believe to record something of the pioneering efforts which in 1947 established the Yale Program of Prepared Childbirth, for at that time it was something of a bold enterprise to allow husbands to be with their wives in a private labor room, to put newborn babies at the mother's bedside, and to use nurse-midwives as teachers of nurses and medical students.

This program came into being not through any single discovery or revelation but the effort of a small group of obstetricians and pediatricians in examining the rationale of many hospital practices then in vogue with a view to making childbirth a more satisfying experience for mothers and fathers and thus have greater benefits for the start of family life. Associated with the author in this endeavor were Grover C. Powers, Arthur H. Morse, Frederick W. Goodrich, Kate H. Hyder and Edith B. Jackson. The last named should long be remembered as a great single force in the establishment of hospital rooming-in in America.

A further purpose of this book is to bring into sharper focus new opportunities which face American obstetricians quite in keeping with the high standards which they uphold and the tradition which for two centuries has kept American obstetrics in the forefront as a major medical discipline. It was through the vision of our earliest teachers of obstetrics in the 18th century and extending to those of the 19th, that the care of women in childbirth by physicians was raised to a new dignity in medical practice.

In considering the expanded maternity care program described in these pages we should recall that the established prenatal program had its most significant growth early in the present century as a result of the combined efforts of obstetricians and public health workers. Today, a like effort by these groups could be productive of greatest good in fostering the concepts that overall maternity care rightfully should be "family centered," that families as well as babies come into being in hospitals, and that an auspicious start for both is of major importance.

FOREWORD

THE invitation to write a foreword to an important book is an honor. But its acceptance carries with it an obligation for honest assessment of the writer and his work. The suggestion of Dr. Thoms that I write a preface to this book carried with it a special appeal. I have been associated with his program of Child Birth With Understanding for many years and in a variety of ways. In the early days I occasionally led a parents' class in discussing care of the newborn. I also participated in the supervisory care provided their babies. Later on as an administrator, I shared some of the responsibility for maintaining the rooming-in part of the project. I use the word "maintaining" advisedly because the program described by Dr. Thoms in this book has not been carried along by its own momentum. It has not always had smooth sailing. There have been skeptics among the hospital administrators, physicians, nurses and even parents who were interested but misinformed about the purposes of the project and its methods. However, this parent and baby care program has become so vital in modern American obstetric and pediatric practice, and so widespread in its use, because of these very people.

Overcoming their initial skepticism through participating in the project, they have uniformly developed such deep feelings of satisfaction that they felt obligated to do everything possible to make such care available to greater numbers of persons facing pregnancy. The appeal to write these words then, is not so much a testimonial to the wisdom, courage and fine human sensitivity of my colleagues, Dr. Herbert Thoms and Dr. Edith Jackson, but more to testify to the fact that parents and persons who worked together in this family-centered approach quite uniformly seemed to have become affected emotionally by the experience. That is, not in a sentimental sense, but more in the deeply moving effect which certain special human relationships bring to people.

I like to believe that the work of Dr. Thoms and his associates has an influence in setting up solid foundations in family relationships; that the focus on the family with opportunities for apprenticeship in baby care by both parents in a milieu which is physically protective and emotionally supportive to mother and child alike, serves as a protective hedge against those forces in our society which seem to be attempting to dissolve the family. There are those who predict that the family will lose its importance as the matrix in which character is molded, anl that family life will become a decorative incident in the system of our society. I would like to believe that this will not come about despite the evidence that in some societies children are more or less forcibly taken from their homes and brought up by the State. It seems to me that the instinct of parental love is so intimately associated with our nature that we will not permit it to ever die out, or even to be threatened with extinction in this way.

There is a variety of evidence which shows that a pregnant woman's outlook upon the world changes as she approaches the time of delivery. Forces which she has not felt before and will not feel until she is pregnant again operate in subtle ways and prepare her emotionally to meet the needs of her child. Much may be done to influence a woman's capacity for motherhood, one of the most important of which is helping her to experience a sense of achievement in delivering her baby and in successfully caring for it in the neonatal period. A woman does not become a mother merely by giving birth to a child; motherhood comes out of a highly personal contact with children and out of carrying responsibly the difficult role of caring for a child. It is in the newborn period that the child needs particular care and nourishment, and responds best in all matters, if he has an opportunity for close contact with his mother. The mother also has needs, the chief of which are encouragement and the opportunity to fall in love with her baby through close contact with it.

It is now that the father too begins to play an important role. Biologically he should have instinctive feelings of pride in his child and affection for his wife. Too often he is relegated to a minor role. In the program championed by Dr. Thoms, both mother and father are encouraged to play the important roles nature has assigned them. The advantage of the rooming-in arrangement is that it permits an apprenticeship for the mother and father in infant care. This not only gives them confidence, but encourages the development of a feeling of kinship with their offspring which makes the stresses of parenthood and baby care less difficult, and so pleasurable that the months and years ahead are approached with self-confidence and joy.

Dr. Thoms has made no exaggerated claims and taken no undeserved credit in presenting the historical and clinical account of his years of experience with the family-centered maternity care at Yale. He would be the first to say that the results of any program aimed at helping human beings are not readily measurable with scientific objectivity. The words "family" and "children" carry a high emotional charge to which most of us respond with strong feelings according to our temperaments and to the experiences we have enjoyed or suffered in our own families. And so it is quite impossible to approach the task of interpretation of the results of this work with a completely open mind and with dispassionate intellectual appraisal. However, it is my belief that the claims presented are neither distorted nor presented with an evangelical enthusiasm. To me this is an account by a compassionate clinician of his many years of work with human beings in which he has demonstrated practically how childbirth and infant care may be provided in a comprehensive fashion which insures the best of medical care, and yet preserves those age-old traits of love and human kindness.

MILTON J. E. SENN, M.D.
Sterling Professor of Pediatrics and Psychiatry
Yale University

CONTENTS

CHILDBIRTH—WITH UNDERSTANDING

I

FIRST CONSIDERATIONS

T HIS book is written for all who have interest in learning about recent developments in obstetrical care which emphasize that childbirth is a body function which should be a more satisfying and educational experience for mothers and fathers. The observations expressed here for the most part emanate from the author's experience in a prepared childbirth and rooming-in program which was started in 1947 at the Yale-New Haven Medical Center under the auspices of the departments of Obstetrics and Gynecology and Pediatrics.

The effect of the emotions on pregnancy and childbirth most certainly was known in ancient times by those who attended women in these functions. They are well expressed in modern times by an American obstetrician named S. C. Bussey who wrote in 1888, "The manifestations of suffering are more influenced by mental and emotional than physical conditions. Delicate and feeble women often pass through the travail of labor with composure and heroism whilst the robust and healthy often exhibit their suffering in the most exaggerated manner. . . . The confidence of the patient in the qualifications of her attendant obviates many emotional disturbances, conducive to the harmonious succession of physiological phenomena. . . ." A noted authority in our day Dr. Helene Deutsche has this to say, "If the disturbing elements within and without are well mastered, if the delivery follows a normal, natural course, and if by direct emotional influences or other means the excess of fear and pain is successfully reduced, childbirth is the greatest and most gratifying experience of women, perhaps of human beings."

Health education has made extraordinary progress in our time but with it little has been done to educate women for their supreme

3

role in childbirth. A very pointed question is asked by Helen Heardman in her book, *A Way to Natural Childbirth,*[3] "How is it that we have allowed women whose function is the reproduction of the race by muscular effort, to embark upon the heavy muscular effort of labour without even a second of real training, and in *fear?"*

"NATURAL CHILDBIRTH"

In recent years as the practice of obstetrics has moved en masse to our hospitals some important aspects of the start of family life seem to have been lost. Some of these lost things are worth while trying to recapture and a number of our obstetrical leaders are endeavoring to do just that. One way is through education for childbirth about which Professor F. J. Browne of the University of London wrote in 1948,[4] "Nothing has been more remarkable in the practice of obstetrics within the past ten years than the increasing appreciation of the value of principles enunciated by Edmund Jacobson in 1929 in his book, *Progressive Relaxation,* and afterward applied to midwifery by Grantly Dick Read in his two books, *Natural Childbirth* and *Revelations of Childbirth."*

Our own experience with this type of approach began in 1947 when a young woman having her first child came to our clinic and said that she had read Dick Read's *Natural Childbirth* and wished to try it. We were willing that she should do so and subsequently witnessed her complete success. Within the next six months 16 other mothers who had expressed a similar desire were all delivered with what support we could then give and their perfomances were highly impressive to members of our staff.

This new interest shortly found for us a friend and supporter in the Maternity Center Association of New York and under their auspices the English physiotherapist, Mrs. Helen Heardman spent several weeks with us applying her methods of muscular control and relaxation to mothers in labor and in addition teaching her techniques to members of our nursing staff. What we now speak of as Prepared Childbirth had its beginning at Yale with Mrs. Heardman as a result of our impressions of what she could do for women in labor.

In our further pursuit of the subject another great boon came to us from the Maternity Center Association who furnished funds for the support of two of their nurse-midwives and a resident physician, all as additions to our regular staff and which continued for a two year period beginning January 1, 1948. The first report of our experience with this better regulated program came later in that year when Dr. F. W. Goodrich and myself reported results in 156 mothers who had their first babies under the regime. In conculsion we stated,[5] "Natural Childbirth is a definite entity which can be taught successfully in a teaching ward service. We believe that natural childbirth technics offer decided advantages to mother and child and are psychologically desirable for most women."

NATURAL CHILDBIRTH IN A TEACHING CLINIC

The idea that these technics could be part of the regular teaching of obstetrics in a medical school was also the subject of a paper of mine entitled, "Natural Childbirth in a Teaching Clinic" which appeared in the *Journal of Obstetrics and Gynaecology of the British Empire* in February 1949. The concluding paragraphs remain unchanged as far as I am concerned and they are repeated here; "In all cases we are careful not to institute relaxation until the patient needs it, and in slow or unduly prolonged labour we do not hesitate to give a sedative if we think the patient needs a period of rest. In the very few cases in which we have found it necessary to use forceps to complete delivery we have used pudendal block anaesthesia, which preserves consciousness at delivery, a thing which these patients seem ardently to desire."

"Among the advantages of natural childbirth are the following; 1. Most of the labours are spontaneous. Because of this, haemorrhage, damage to maternal soft parts, and foetal morbidity and mortality have a low incidence. 2. Certain risks attendant on the use of anaesthetic methods are avoided. 3. The psychological advantage to the patient is very real. An immediate and close bond is established between the mother and her baby, which in the opinion of psychiatrists who have observed natural childbirth establishes an important mother-child relaionship which can have a deep and lasting effect. 4. The advantage from the standpoint of a teaching clinic may be summarized by saying that natural childbirth from the start of indoctrination to the discharge of the patient offers an opportunity to teach young doctors, nurses and medical students that childbirth is a truly physiological process to be considered without fear or anxiety, to be conducted with utmost skill and understanding, and to be regarded as worthy of the finest efforts of the medical and nursing profession."

"In conclusion, I believe that the techniques of natural childbirth can be taught in a teaching hospital, that it offers decided physical and psychological advantages to mother and child, and that the technique recommended deserves further study to the end that it may become a part of every antenatal programme."

In the early years of our program we referred to it as the Natural Childbirth Program. This was an inheritance from Dr. Dick Read and Mrs. Heardman whose books used these words in titles. It was not long before we realized that the term "natural childbirth" was unfortunate because it suggested to many people, including writers for magazines, that in primitive cultures childbirth was essentially painless and that in someway it could be transferred into our own, two gross errors. The fact is, that labor in primitive peoples is not regularly a painless event in spite of a wide spread impression. Clelland Ford in his *Comparative Study of Reproduction* says,[7] "The popular impression of childbirth in primitive society as painless and easy is definitely contradicted by our cases. Fear of a difficult and painful labor motivates women in all societies to follow strict rules during pregnancy." Again, one but has to look at the illustrations in Engelmann's classic *Labor Among Primitive Peoples,* (St. Louis, 1888) to see something of the horrors inflicted through ignorance in difficult labor in these women.

THE PREPARED CHILDBIRTH PROGRAM

In definition, the Prepared Childbirth Program at Yale emphasizes that childbirth is a natural body process and that it is important for the expectant mother to learn that bringing her baby into the world is a cooperative endeavor in which she plays the most important role. It is also of high importance that her attendants have some insight into her psychological needs and a first hand knowledge of the details of the Program, of what is good support during labor and of efficient after-care, including rooming-in.

In these first considerations it is important to say a few words about anesthesia methods in the program. None of the important writers on natural childbirth have ever claimed that childbirth should be conducted without anesthetic aid. According to Dick Read,[8] "Pain is the only justification; it does not matter whether the pain is secondary to fear or whether it is primarily physical."

Dr. C. D. Davis characterizes the present program at Yale as,[9] "Education of the mother and father, exercises, relaxation, reduction in amount of anesthesia and analgesia, support during labor and rooming-in, all aimed at helping physicians to be better obstetricians. It is not possible to weigh objectively the relative values of the various facets of the Prepared Childbirth Program." He also points out that the obstetrician may not be in an ideal position to evaluate the whole story because he only sees the middle of the book. What the mother's parental relationships were, what her marriage is and what is her feminine role cannot be learned in a few short office visits. What is equally discouraging is that when the baby is born and the pediatrician takes over the obstetrician, "has the book taken away from him and he must be satisfied with another single chapter in yet another book."

With the almost complete hospitalization of childbirth in America it becomes obvious that our hospitals at present have programs of procedure in order to insure safety for mother and child. The addition of such things as continuous labor support and rooming-in interferes in no way with this objective but actually augments the effort. The hospital, too, has now become the place of birth of the family unit and whether this gets off to an auspicious start may depend to no small extent on the adequacy of the professional care, the influence of environmental forces and the impressions left in the minds of the new parents. What the obstetrician's role in all this is has been wisely commented upon by Dr. T. L. Montgomery in a presidential address given in 1955 before the American Association of Obstetricians and Gynecologists in which he said,[10] "Yet perhaps it is time that a few here and there begin to think about conserving—conserving in general—as well as in obstetrics, about saving things that were at one time considered worth while; minds that are clear to think, families that are a unit of strength, ideals that children may be raised by, homespun virtues which lead the individual to do for others as he would be done by."

"Over a period of years the feeling has grown upon me that the obstetrician has more to do with all this than he has any concept. In his profession he treats with the beginnings of life and the circumstances which surround them, his influence in the home is second only to that of the family doctor with whom he may often be embodied. How he handles the course of pregnancy, the progress in labor, and the procedures of delivery; how he draws together the family around the advent of the newborn may exert more influence upon the future of the race, for good or for evil, than any one other individual may bring to bear. . . . Concerning the emotional factors which surround the function of reproduction and which our psychiatric friends speak of, we are prone to scoff. I suspect we would all agree, however, that for the two patients concerned in obstetric practice, birth has tremendous significance; to the mother it is the most important event physically and emotionally that she will face in her entire life; to the baby quite independent of other considerations, it is the most critical physiological development which the new organism will have to make in its entire existence."

A WIDER OUTLOOK

A Prepared Childbirth Program, such as described herein, must be considered as still in the nature of an experiment and capable of further development. The type of instruction, the extent of husband participation, the clinic and hospital environment, the kind of support during labor, rooming-in procedures, and the economics involved, all are subjects for discussion. There are, however, two aspects of our program which I consider to be paramount in good obstetrics everywhere, proper support during labor and rooming-in for mothers who want it. Our experience in these and other matters is given in detail in later chapters.

Finally, it would be well for obstetricians to read again the words of T. L. Montgomery previously quoted. The reproduction of the race and the start of family life have heavy responsibilities for them and for all who are concerned in maternity care. In the words of Samuel H. Miller, "There is no man so poverty stricken that he does not have in his experience certain circumstances where life literally broke open, the superficial surface of it was breached, and the mystery and glory of it like a great tide lifted him from the flats and shallows of mean existence."[11] One such experience is the advent of a newborn baby the reality of which has made the heart of man responsive all through the eon of his existence.

REFERENCES

1. Bussey, S. C.: *American System of Obstetrics.* Lea Brothers, Philadelphia, 1888, p. 486.

2. Deutsche H.: *The Psychology of Women.* Grune & Stratton Inc., New York, 1945.

3. Heardman, H.: *A Way to Natural Childbirth.* Williams and Wilkins Co., Baltimore, 1948.

4. Browne, F. J.: Foreword in H. Heardman's, *A Way to Natural Childbirth.* Baltimore, 1948.

5. Goodrich, F. W., Jr. and Thoms, H.: A Clinical Study of Natural Childbirth. *American J. Obstetrics & Gynecology,* v. 56, p. 875, 1948.

6. Thoms, H.: Natural Childbirth in a Teaching Clinic. *J. Obst. & Gyn.,* British Empire v. 56, p. 19, 1949.

7. Ford, C. S.: Comparative Study of Human Reproduction. Yale Anthropological Series, No. 52, Yale University Press. 1945.

8. Dick Read, G.: *Childbirth without Fear.* Harper & Brothers, New York, 1944.

9. Davis, C. D.: *Prepared Childbirth.* Section II, Chapter 23. v. 1, p. 85, C. H. Davis' System of Obstetrics and Gynecology.

10. Montgomery, T. L.: President's Address. American Association of Obstetricians and Gynecologists. *Am. J. Obstetrics & Gynecology,* v. 71, p. 469, 1956.

11. Miller, S. H.: *The Great Realities,* Harper & Brothers, New York, 1955, p. 99.

II

WE CAN DO BETTER

SOME leaders in obstetrics today are questioning certain procedures in conventional maternity care. This sign of growth is to be welcomed even though some barriers to change seem formidable. Chief of these is said to be the "obstetric load" doctors and nurses are called upon to carry under present circumstances. Many authorities agree, however, that with better organization and a more spread out effort changes can be made. Many patients during the long hours of labor do not need a doctor in close attendance but can be administered to by skillful if less highly trained persons. Even when assembly line methods are necessary for efficiency in operation there is no need for them to be impersonal. There are efficiently run large hotels which still remain friendly and to an extent homelike places. Women in maternity hospitals are not sick but well people. They too can be considered and treated, as guests.

OBSTETRICS AS PREVENTIVE MEDICINE

As early as 1939, Dr. John S. Fairbairn of London, called for a wider outlook in obstetrics, saying,[1] "Midwifery with its pre- and post-maternity clinics, comprises the early links in the chain of services aiming at the betterment of the health and physique of the rising generation. . . . There is not any other clinical subject which can equal that of maternity and child welfare in the opportunities for the education of students in the assessment and maintenance of normal health and the principles and practice of the prevention of disease." Fairbairn calls for further efforts to discover the mother's reaction to her pregnancy, "as it and other factors effect the management of her pregnancy and labour by measures being taken to remove those that might interfere with normal function."

Dr. John Bowley, of the Tavistock Health Clinic in London,

10

wrote in 1950,[2] "Numerous studies have made it quite clear that when a child is deprived of maternal care his development is retarded physically, emotionally, and socially. Let us reflect for a moment on the astonishing practice which has been followed in maternity wards of separating mothers and babies immediately after birth and ask ourselves whether this is the way to promote a mother-child relationship?" In this same year, *Briefs,* a publication of the Maternity Center Association of New York reported,[3] "A clash has arisen in recent years between consumers of medical care, with their searching demand for family and individual security, and the suppliers of that care. The root of that clash is found in the attitude of mind of many of the people who provide care, from the hospital board member to the receptionist in the clinic. Many of these people do not recognise that a change of mind is taking place among the consumers. The care provided in too many hospitals is not in harmony with the findings of psychosomatic medicine and the relationship of the emotions to physical health and all of this to sound, happy family living and the development of healthy personality."

ANALGESIA AND ANESTHESIA IN OBSTETRICS

Some facts in this aspect of obstetrics need airing. Dr. C. L. Buxton of Yale, speaking in 1956 before the Medical Society of the State of New York told that audience,[4] "From 1934 until the present, innumerable articles have appeared in the obstetric literature describing successes or failures with innumerable kinds of analgesia and anesthesia. This has represented a very definite attitude of mind on the part of the obstetrician. This attitude is expressed by one of the most experienced and capable users of obstetrical analgesia when he says, 'the ultimate object (of analgesia) is a creation of complete amnesia without affecting the course of labor.'" But, Dr. Buxton points out, statistics attest to the fact that such an attitude is not without considerable danger for some alarming figures bear this out. Thus, in 1952 in New York City, anesthesia was the cause of maternal mortality in fifth place behind hemorrhage, infection, toxemia and heart disease. In Nashville during an eight year period the mortality from anesthesia led one reporter to call it "the fourth horseman of the obstetrical apocalypse." Fitzgerald and Webster reporting in 1953, found that 44 per cent of all maternal deaths in three St. Louis hospitals were from anesthesia. Considering these and other reports, Buxton says, "Aside from the above mentioned anesthesia hazards; the disadvantage of this technique (complete amnesia) from a physical point of view lay in the frequent restlessness and intractibility of the mother and the narcotized baby who nevertheless could be made to respond fairly adequately to stimulus within a reasonable time after delivery. There has been a gradually increasing awareness, possibly stimulated by obstetric patients themselves, that the psychologic reaction on the part of the woman to complete amnesia during labor and delivery, frequently was one of great dissatisfaction, frustration and unhappiness. In our humane and charitable attempt to relieve her of pain—we may possibly have deprived her of something even more important—her own profound and stimulating satisfaction in the awareness of her contribution to humanity."

More recently from across the sea (1960) comes the voice of another professor of obstetrics, Dr. Norman Morris of the University of London. In "Human Relations in Obstetrical Practice" appearing in *The Lancet,* he says our present hospital system often fails miserably in its care of the patient's emotions, that the feeling of personal achievement is lost, drowned in a sea of inhumanity. Accordingly,[5] "Women attend antenatal clinics regularly, often as many as fourteen times. The clinic is usually drab and colorless, painted a bottle green, brown or dirty cream. There are rows of uncomfortable benches. There is an atmosphere of coldness, unfriendliness and severity more in keeping with the spirit of an income tax office. The clinic is often over crowded, at best, a crude appointment system is in operation. Despite this, women often wait one to three hours. The interview itself is usually extremely brief and under such conditions there is little encouragement for the patient to ask questions or relieve herself of any nagging fears or doubts. Therefore she often remains in gross ignorance of what is happening to her. The doctors and nurses also remain virtual strangers since she rarely sees the same one at each visit. Doctors interviewing large numbers of women on an endless conveyor belt system inevitably lose their sensitivity. . . . When the patient arrives at the hospital in labor she usually goes through a ceremonial known as being admitted. Before this ceremonial can begin she often has to supply some particulars to the porter or nurse on duty. She is then undressed, shaved, given an enema and hot bath. When this ritual is completed, the patient either goes into a first stage labor ward or into a general ward."

"In the first stage ward, usually a large room with several beds, there are often many women in different stages of labor. To a woman early in labor, it is extremely frightening to be brought into such close constant with women in the later stages of labor who may appear distressed and upset."

Dr. Morris also asks some very pertinent questions such as, why is there so little thought for the mother as an individual? How far is this situation the end result of poor training and can it be prevented? Is this unsympathetic attitude a form of defense mechanism against the constant load of anxiety in every maternity unit? Nurses in training always seem to be walking about and are seldom encouraged to sit down and talk with their patients. Does this also contribute to a later development of an inhuman attitude? Why do some hospital doctors appear cold and distant? Do obstetricians in training have enough opportunity to learn much about normal labor and do they develop much insight into women as women? Has the physician-accoucheur been replaced by the surgeon-accoucheur with little interest in normal labor? Do some nurses and doctors find childbirth repugnant and not something wonderful?"

WE CAN DO BETTER

Dr. Morris has answers to some of his questions and they interest us for many of his problems are our own." We must get rid of that awful method," he writes, "of dividing patients into cooperative or uncooperative, into easy or difficult. We must insure that no patient is ever at the mercy of a midwife's own frustration and mixed up emotions. No senior sister must be allowed to exert her authority by means of a reign of terror, to which even the consultant obstetrician must sometimes submit. . . . A new approach is needed and in that we must plan our maternity units so that they reflect joy rather than sorrow, hope rather than gloom, life rather than death. Somehow we must try to reproduce in the hospital the natural tranquility that often develops quite spontaneously with home confinements. Architects must combine with us to experiment in new forms of design. . . . If we could see pregnancy as a time of preparation not only for labor but for all that family life means, and if we can make childbirth a more positive experience then I think social repercussions will be remarkable. . . . The next century will undoubtedly see a great advance in our understanding of all the complex factors that influence and govern human relationships. The health, happiness and possibly the survival of our children will depend on the success of our studies in this field."

A courageous and timely editorial on Morris's indictment of present day obstetrical practice in our hospitals comes from the *Midwives Chronicle* and influential British publication which says,[6] "Do we not tend to lose sight of the fact that our responsibility includes not only the duty of foreseeing, preventing and treating physical hazards; but also the obligations to carry out these clinical functions in a way which does not intrude upon the dignity of our fellow women and detract from the right to feel a sense of joyful accomplishment in what *they* have achieved with what should be our *humble* help? . . . How necessary is hospital routine? Even if we feel, after critical examination, that the discipline is still necessary to maintain a certain *esprit de corps* among the ranks of our professional lives, by what right do we impose it on those whom we serve? . . . We as a profession may be wasting our time pursuing tasks which, having outlasted their original purpose, are now serving to deviate us from our real purpose as midwives, which is to be *with-women*."

In a similar vein, Vera R. Keane[7] reports in *Briefs* (1958) in "From the Patient's Viewpoint," We forget say the mothers that it is *they* who are having the babies and not *us,* and without waiting to find out their real feelings, we impose our own philosophy and viewpoint upon one and all, willy-nilly. Difficulties arise when the parent and the professionals who are assisting her in labor, hold diametrically opposite convictions. What usually happens is that the attendant acts upon his or her feelings, and behaves as though no other viewpoint were sensible, or even possible. In such instances, relief from pain, emotional support, and the assurances of a safe outcome are no longer attainable for the woman in labor."

OUR OWN SHORTCOMINGS

The above criticisms apply with equal force to conditions in our own country. We too, have our drab clinics, our overworked staffs, our harassed attendants, and with characteristic "efficiency" we too, have assembly-line obstetrics as N. J. Eastman the professor of obstetrics at Johns Hopkins has pointed out. He writes,[8] "In view of the huge number of patients which most obstetricians both in clinic and private practice, are called upon to attend these days, and in view of the systematizing of hospital obstetric practices, both medical and nursing, these important psychological aspects are often neglected in favor of what we might call assemby-line methods. Here the mother becomes a case, a hospital number, rather than a person."

Another professor of obstetrics, H. B. Atlee of Halifax, whose wise observations appear throughout this book, says,[9] "Maternity hospitals imitate in sheeplike conformity the procedures and attitudes of general hospitals. The maternity sections of general hospitals are completely dominated by the philosophy of the whole of which they form a part. It is our belief that both should present a different face to the woman in labor from the one presented to the woman with a gall bladder full of stones. The woman in labor is not in a hospital because she has a disease, but in order to carry out in the safest possible milieu that physiological process on which the continuation of the race depends. . . . The more I ponder over what goes on in maternity hospitals, the more I am convinced that some change of attitude is long overdue. With this in mind we have attempted at our hospitals to gear our attitudes and architecture more rationally to the needs and satisfactions of the laboring woman. We have not succeeded fully, or anything like fully. It is very difficult to alter human habits, as the results of 2000 years of Christianity testify. Since it is the nurses more than any other workers, who come into closest and most prolonged contact with the woman, we have tried to impress most earnestly on these our philosophy. . . . We exhort them, not only on behalf of those practising Natural Childbirth, but of all women in labor, to follow this obstetrical golden rule: *Do unto every woman as if you yourself were in labor*. At the same time we are not unmindful that this rule should apply to all maternity hospital workers who come in contact with the woman—including our masculine selves."

My own view of some of these matters I have expressed previously,[10] "Everyone concerned is becoming aware that the implications of maternity care go beyond safeguarding mothers from the hazards of childbirth and extend into the actual care of our evolving civilization. No one can sincerely question the main benefits that change from home to hospital has brought to the childbearing woman. Certain authorities do question the usefulness of some aspects of conventional hospital care. I refer to such practices as separation of the mother and infant in the central nursery system, the use of the general labor room in which the woman in labor is exposed to others in various stages of the process, the inability of a husband to stay with his wife during the long early part of the labor and the heavy use of sedative drugs to obliterate the mother's memory of the experience."

In the use of these amnesic drugs I would add for the sake of the uninformed that their side effects sometimes produce such excitation that for protection patients have to be put in restraint-type beds and other devices used reminiscent of a medieval madhouse. I am confident, however, that the obstetrics of the future will not be practised in any such atmosphere no matter what "ideal" amnesia drug is newly discovered.

It is obvious that the remedy for most of our troubles and shortcomings lies in profesional hands. As doctors and nurses we are going to have to raise our sights in obstetrics to include a consideration of the impact of childbearing on the start of family life. From our experience at New Haven, I can testify that it is possible for an obstetrical clinic to have a rebirth and develop within itself many of the fine attributes extolled by Francis Peabody in his classic, "Soul of the Clinic." We should not have to be reminded that of all clinical divisions in a hospital that of obstetrics has the greatest potential for being a friendly place and a happy one.

REFERENCES

1. Fairbairn, J. S.: Plea for a Wider Outlook in the Teaching of Obstetrics, *J. Obst. & Gyn.*, British Empire v. 46, p. 201, 1939.
2. Bowlby, J.: *Briefs*. Published by Maternity Center Assn. v. xxiii, p. 134.

3. *Briefs.*

4. Buxton, C. L.: An Evaluation of a Prepared Childbirth Program, *New York State J. Medicine,* v. 56, p. 2658, 1956.

5. Morris, N.: Human Relations in Obstetrics. *Lancet* (London), Apr. 23, 1960.

6. Midwives Chronicle and Nursing Notes: June, 1960, v. 24, quoted by *Briefs,* Oct., 1960, p. 153.

7. Keane, V. R.: Maternity Care from the Parent's Viewpoint. *Briefs,* April, 1958, v. 22, p. 56.

8. Eastman, N. J.: *Briefs,* v. 17, 8, 1953-54.

9. Atlee, H. B.: *Natural Childbirth.* Thomas, Springfield, 1956.

10. Thoms, H.: *Our Obstetric Heritage.* The Shoestring Press, Hamden, 1960.

III

THE PREPARED CHILDBIRTH PROGRAM

Many names have been used in connection with a program of obstetric care which emphasizes the psychological aspects of child-bearing and training for the event. Some of these are: Natural Childbirth, Educated Childbirth, Psychoprophylactic Preparation, Training for Childbirth, Prepared Childbirth. I believe the latter term is more inclusive and the most preferable. The Prepared Childbirth Program as it has developed at Yale does recognise that most women in labor do have pain but that there is a great deal of difference in feeling pain as distress and minding it as discomfort. In most instances experience has shown that the prepared mother does feel less pain and is better able to cope with it than the woman who is less informed and therefore often has to cope with anxiety and fear. The prepared woman is coached and trained so that she can relax at the time of painful uterine contractions and also not to anticipate with too much concern. It is certainly unwise and actually harmful for any attendant to try and convince a woman in labor that she is not having pain or to minimize her discomfort. Most of all she needs encouragement in a sympathetic and forthright manner, explanation as to what is happening, to know the progress she is making and to be coached in her efforts to relax. In other words, *skilled support during labor.* Women who have had adequate preparation and who receive such support as a rule will need but a minimum of anesthetic aids and will as a result deliver babies who will need no resusitation whatever.

THE RUSSIAN SYSTEM

Dr. Clarence D. Davis of the Yale Staff has written on the so called psychoprophylactic or Russian system in comparison to that practised at Yale. The former is the "Painless Childbirth" which

Russian obstetricians have exploited so widely. "According to Vellay," says Davis,[1] "psychoprophylaxis is 'verbal analgesia' based on 'rational education of pregnant women.' It uses essentially the therapeutic agent, 'La Parole.' This is the second signal system of Pavlov. It is fundamentally based on the application of conditioned reflex studies and is applied to labor by Soviet obstetricians such as Velvolski, Nicolaiev, etc. The avowed purpose of this technique is to train the mind of the parturient so that she will consider the course of pregnancy and labor to be a chain of conditioned reflexes which can be used during labor and delivery. The pregnant woman thus learns to deliver herself the way a child learns to read and write. She eliminates from her mind all noxious influences and bad recollections of labor which have been previously encountered and which might inhibit her mind in the development of the above conditioned reflexes. She should have mental control so that she can direct and regulate the functions of her body during the process of parturition. By no stretch of the imagination does the Prepared Childbirth Program as it is practiced at Yale work by any such devious mechanism."

There has been a considerable interest on the part of some as to whether hypnotism plays a part in labor support. One writer states that a state of "waking hypnotism" is produced. Another, that the labor experience is a masochistic one in which the woman weaves pain together with the act of parturition so that pain does not stand out as an isolated reaction but becomes part of a pleasurable experience. So it is that all sorts of speculations and theories now find their way into the obstetric literature. They will not be discussed further in this book.

GRANTLY DICK READ IN NEW HAVEN

On January 22, 1947, Dr. Dick Read made a short visit to New Haven and spoke before a group of medical students and nurses. His remarks at that time were recorded and transcribed. They tell something of his methods and of himself as a forceful and engaging personality. The following are excerpts; "With respect to childbirth it is generally accepted as unpleasant business. A woman does not expect to have a baby without some discomfort. Frequently she does not know much about this job she is to do. She wants a baby but doesn't want to *have* it. . . . Why should this thing be painful? Especially when you think further that for the race childbirth is essential. A woman is constructed for this purpose. Undoubtedly every emotional experience in the life of the average healthy woman is one of a natural urge stemming from childhood through puberty. In one way or another, nature urges her toward mating. Marriage for her is a great and natural thing and home building makes her life really worth living. When she becomes pregnant she builds up her womanhood, changing from a girl to a woman. Then she is TOLD; what is she told? For generations, what has she been told? By what association in her thinking is she able to look forward to bearing a child?"

"I am unwilling to believe that nature is going to lead the females of our race through life, giving them everything which is beautiful, everything which is satisfying and desirable in a woman's life from the standpoint of sex and then turn around and say, 'Thank you very much. You have my course of events most excellently. You are now a grown woman and about to complete your purpose and I am going to give you absolute Hell for it. Tell me, if you can see any sense in that or what law of nature justifies it. We have got to find out why this happens and whether it is reasonable. . . . So, we set about educating our patients a bit telling them; 'In spite of the Bible, in spite of your maiden aunts, in spite of what your friends say, it is all wrong. They speak of you in hushed whispers, they give you a blessing and say they will be relieved when you come through all right. . . . The teaching of young women of things relating to any horrors of childbirth is one of the most criminal things in Western society. I have called it the 'fifth column of the Devil,' because it is true. . . . Our education of women in eliminating fear proved to be reasonably successful . . . I started gradually, teaching them that they were beautifully made for having a baby, how large the child was at the various months, what they might expect in labor. Also about expecting the movements of the baby and when they knew what it was the baby became a part of their minds. This kept them in touch with what was happening, made them thrill with the idea and not be afraid of it. . . . You must not allow a woman to have any anxiety on her mind. There must be created within her a background of her obstetric presence which can never entertain a doubt. I tell her why this education is important and teach her physical exercises. About labor, she is not told that it is easy. At the time of labor I tell her, 'Look here, this is a day of pretty hard work. It requires threefold fundamental virtues. Show yourself and me, whether you happen to be possessed of them. They are, patience, control, and the ability to work hard when called upon.' . . . The intelligence of pregnant women is very interesting. They all have a level of obstetric intelligence which is the same in all classes. And, all of them can pick up a knowledge of pregnancy, labor and delivery if it is put to them clearly. But, there is no call to portray to a patient how brilliant you are. You cannot deceive her. She may pretend and act if she believes you but it will be mere acting out of a sense of protection. . . .

"The value of the exercises is in the simple act of relaxation. . . . Proper respiration is the first principle of relaxation. . . . When a child is born there are "three labors" and you must have perfect knowledge of all three if you wish a woman to have her child according to the laws of nature. First, there is the purely mechanical labor, secondly, the labor of the woman at the emotional level and third, the labor of the attendant of the woman, the most dangerous of all. . . . The emotional labor is the most important of the three and it is dramatically different in the first and second stages."

It is the custom in some places when the outlet stretches a bit to hurry labor along and wind it up. I do not like an obstetrician who is dogmatic about principles; such a one has a limited field of knowledge. From those whom you differ most you will learn most. . . . The obstetrician is the man who stands by with a purpose, but he is not the man who must assume that his genius has called upon him to improve upon the works of God."

PREPARED CHILDBIRTH AT YALE

The Prepared Childbirth Program at Yale has two chief aspects. (1) The Mothers' Classes. (2) Support During Labor. All mothers who register at the University Clinic division of the hospital are told about the program by a clinic nurse. Many private patients of doctors of the University and General Staffs are informed about the program by their physicians. Program participants are therefore on a self-selection basis. This, of course, favors good patient cooperation. Mothers do not begin classes until about the middle months of pregnancy and there are usually about five series going making it easier for mothers to arrange their time. The mothers' classes are conducted by specially trained nurses and nurse-mid-wives. Each class is made up of not more than twenty women. Aids in teaching include the blackboard, The Maternity Center Birth Atlas, lantern slides and the showing of a motion picture. The principles of pregnancy and labor are taught and informal discussion encouraged. The limitation to small groups tends to establish an air of informality and to promote discussion. Sometimes classes are attended by "repeat" mothers who in a second pregnancy wish to brush up on the technics. They are welcome additions and often are of considerable help in clearing away self-consciousness on the part of the neophytes.

The exercise technics which are taught are aimed at muscular control, body relaxation, abdominal breathing and correction of posture. The final class in each series includes a tour of the labor and delivery rooms where the anesthesia apparatus can be seen and explained. Husbands are invited to attend this tour. In addition to mother's classes evening classes are held for husbands and wives. These are given by an obstetrician and a pediatrician. The former talks about the physiology of pregnancy and labor and the latter discusses the newborn and rooming-in. Discussions also follow these sessions which are limited to two hours for each one.

The course material for the mothers' classes includes the following subjects.

1. *Introduction to Pregnancy*
    Growth of the embryo.
    Anatomy and physiology of the generative organs.
2. *Adapation*
    Adaptation to pregnancy.
    Signs and symptoms during each trimester period.
3. *Diet during Pregnancy*
4. *Labor*
    Onset—signs and symptoms.
    Stages of labor.

Physiology of labor.

Progress of labor.

5. *Delivery*

The process of delivery.

Review of the stages of labor.

6. *Postpartum Care—Rooming-in*

7. *Breast Care* (Optional).

8. *Baby Care* (Optional)

The above outline of course material is based on that described by Dr. Davis referred to above.

In her book *Family-Centered Maternity Nursing,* Ernestine Wiedenbach of our staff emphasizes that "The advantage of group conferences lies in the social atmosphere, the support and encouragement members give each other and the range of information covered through discussions as a result of the varied interests and experiences of members of the group. . . . As a rule the social, economic or educational status of the individual members is of less concern to the mothers or parents in the group than the interest they all have in common, i.e., the coming of their babies."

Miss Wiedenbach also says, "Conferences seem to be more meaningful when they are in discussion rather than in lecture form, geared to the mothers' or parents' interest and understanding but within the framework of an organized plan. Discussions with a series, for instance, may form on such subjects as: (1) Physiology of childbearing, including concepts of how the baby grows, develops and is born. (2) Progressive changes during pregnancy and adjustments which the mother may make to promote comfort, health and hygiene. (3) Nutrition—what to eat and why, and how to prepare the food. (4) Concepts of labor—progressive physiological development and its implications. (5) Team action during labor,— the role of the mother and the father, and a rehearsal for the event. (6) The day of the baby's arrival—When to come to the hospital, what to take, where to go, what to expect and what to do. (Note) Added interest and meaning are often given to this discussion when it is preceded by a tour of the hospital's obstetric department, in particular the labor and delivery rooms."

The plan which Miss Wiedenbach follows in classwork may occupy 50 minutes, followed by a ten minute intermission which precedes the exercise period, the whole lasting two hours.

THE EXERCISES

The exercises are fully described in my book *Understanding Natural Childbirth* as well as in Miss Wiedenbach's and others. They will be but summarized here. They consist of techniques of breath control and the understanding of certain body mechanics aimed at relaxation to relieve tension and anxiety. Classes in these exercises are usually started in the fourth or fifth month of pregnancy at a time when the pregnancy is well established in the mother's mind as well as in her body. Patients of private physicians are only accepted on written request by the doctor who obviously must be aware of what the classwork is like and its aims. The advantages to him are numerous especially in the type of labor-support he can count on and the cooperation of his patient within her capabilities.

As I have stated elsewhere in this book I believe the classwork for mothers and fathers can with profit include more parenthood preparation. In the present chapter emphasis has been placed chiefly on the teaching of the physiology of pregnancy and labor and the exercises. The best way, and perhaps the only way, for a doctor or nurse to get a complete grasp of the program with a view to teaching or directing something similar is to attend such classes as a spectator and see at first hand their operation. The relegation of classwork to a staff member who is inexperienced or not interested will not have results desired. As Dr. Dick Read has pointed out, the audience of such a lecturer will not be deceived even though they are polite.

RESULTS

In a paper published in 1955, I recorded certain results of our program with conclusions. It is in part here reproduced:

Certain results related to the program lend themselves easily to statistical analysis, others cannot be evaluated so readily. These can be referred to as the qualitative results, and are as real and as important as the quantitative. In any program evaluation a control series of patients can render valuable information but such a study cannot be carried out easily in an institution using the same staff of doctors and nurses for both groups. In our early experience we endeavored to make a study of results in prepared and unprepared mothers. The data which were gathered furnished much interesting information but a truer perspective would have been obtained if separate staff attendants had been used, preferably on separate wards.

Satisfactory control studies have been carried out as in the report to me by Helen Heardman just previous to her death. These were the findings in 1,000 women, 500 trained according to her system of preparation (average attendance at class, 8.4 times) and 500 controls none of whom had any specific training. All of the women were supposedly primigravidas. The series was taken from ten voluntary hospitals and various nursing homes under the care of consultants. The average length of labor in the trained group was 17 hours, 10 minutes; controls 20 hours, 42 minutes. Forceps deliveries; trained group 47, controls 86. Postpartum hemorrhage; trained group nine, controls 15.

Certain of our results habe been published from time to time and recently we reviewed the deliveries in 2,000 women,[5] 1,000 of whom were delivered between January 1, 1949 and March 31, 1950 and a second group of 1,000 women delivered between October 1, 1950 and March 30, 1952. A brief summary is here given. It is offered for possible comparison with results in clinics where a similar type of program is not followed.

TYPE OF DELIVERY

	Primigravidas	Multigravidas
Spontaneous birth 1,761 (88.1 per cent)	550	1,211
Operative (total), 239 (11.9 per cent)	153	86
Vaginal operative, 166 (8.3 per cent)	122	44
Cesarean section, 73 (3.6 per cent)	31	42

ANALGESIA AND ANESTHESIA, 1927
VAGINAL DELIVERIES

Analgesia. No analgesia was given in 660 deliveries or in 34.2 per cent. A single dose of demerol or seconal (not more than 125 mgm.) was given in 1,195 deliveries or 62.0 per cent.

Anesthesia. In 562 women (29.1 per cent) no second stage anesthetic was given. In 1,275 women (66.1 per cent) second stage anesthesia was limited to intermittent trilene or nitrous oxide inhalations.

In 123 women a major type of anesthesia, either general or spinal was given, these include those delivered by cesarean section.

RESULTS FOR THE INFANT
2,024 infants delivered (1,500 gms. or over)

Antenatal infant deaths 18
Intranatal infant deaths 8
Neonatal infant deaths 4

A total of 30 infant deaths in 2,000 deliveries.

In addition to the above figures we have a greatly lessened number of depressed infants at birth, in fact it is a rare occurrence even in slight degrees. There is a decrease in the length of labors, 52.7 per cent of the total delivered within six hours and 49.0 per cent of the primigravidas in less than ten hours. We have less operative deliveries, less blood loss, happier mothers, and parents better adjusted to the start of family life.

Of the 2,000 women in this study many attended the full course of antenatal classes, others some, and a good proportion none. Of these latter the majority were multigravidas who may have attended classes with previous confinements, or could not give the time to it, or were not interested. However, all of the women who were delivered vaginally were given the supportive techniques during labor and delivery and those who desired rooming-in for themselves and their babies usually could be accommodated.

ECONOMICS

This aspect of the subject suggests a question. Is the added effort and expense of the program warranted? There is no question that the effort involves an expenditure of more time on the part of doctors and nurses in both obstetric and pediatric care. Doctors in both groups conduct parents' classes, an experience which thus far has been for them a welcome assignment. In the labor and delivery rooms the physician in charge probably gives more time in supervising the support of the patient.

The chief economic problem relates to nursing service. This involves the teaching of mothers' classes and the support of the patient in labor. Without doubt these activities and certain rooming-in procedures are developing new fields of endeavor in obstetric and pediatric nursing. In similar programs carried out in Great Britain the use of the trained physiotherapist for some of these duties seems to be giving satisfaction. Some developments along this line have been started in this country.

In our program a source of income is derived from the mothers' classes. A moderate fee is paid by all who register for the course except those belonging in the ward status. Many women in the classes are patients of private practitioners who desire this type of instruction for their expectant mothers.

In evaluating the worth of the program we must consider not only our statistical results but the increased satisfaction of the mothers and fathers. These are satisfactions which find reflection in the efforts of those who share the program responsibilities.

OTHER RESULTS

Dr. H. B. Atlee in 1956[6] published some early results of his program of Natural Childbirth at the Department of Obstetrics and Gynecology at Dalhousie University in Halifax. These resulted from a study of 1200 women and separated into three main categories; (1) the performance of the woman in labor; (2) her sense of achievement and satisfaction; (3) the effects on the baby.

Performance of the Woman

According to Dr. Atlee, this was greatly influenced by, (1) the amount of pain she seemed to feel; (2) the length of labor; (3) by the support she received in the hospital from nurses, doctors, husbands, etc. A considerable number of the 1200 women did not get the full support that might have been available or that was available to others in the series. Accordingly, says Dr. Atlee,[6] "Our results merely show what can be done in any hospital where a minimum of training is undertaken, and no additional nursing staff available."

TABLE 1

NATURE OF PERFORMANCE

Category	Sedative	Anesthetic	Labor Type	Will Repeat
Excellent	None	Local	Spontaneous	Yes
Very Good	One only	Local	Spontaneous	Yes
Good	1 or 2	Local & Trilene	Mostly Spontaneous	Yes
Helped	one or more	General or Spinal	Mostly Forceps	Yes
Failure	Got no apparent help whatsoever and will not repeat.			

TABLE 2

PERFORMANCE FIGURES

Performance	Primiparae	Multiparae
Excellent	26%	46%
Very Good	22%	11%
Good	28%	18%
Helped	22%	18%
Failures	8%	7%

In his summary Dr. Atlee comments, "We got the impression that some women were not actually feeling pain as we know it in cases not doing Natural Childbirth. This seemed to be so in a considerable number of those in the *Excellent* category. In others there was pain, but the woman seemed to have developed the capacity to bear it and seemed satisfied to bear it. What we do notice as doctors and nurses, is the extra-ordinary emotional control shown by these women as compared with those not undertaking the method. Much of the tumult and shouting that previously characterized our Case Room has died. Whether they are having pain or not the women who are using this method put on a much better show—and appear to take considerable pride in doing so. "In Sense of Achievement and Satisfactions, Dr. Atlee says, "Ninety per cent of our women were more or less enthusiastic about the regime, and about the same percentage would repeat it. . . . The use of Natural Childbirth has cut down the incidence of prophylactic forceps. Whereas this type of application is done in 30 per cent of all private deliveries in our hospital it was done in 18 percent of our total group of Natural Childbirthers, and in only 12 per cent of those practicing it more faithfully. Some of us feel that even this incidence is higher than it really need be."

Effect on Baby

Under this Category Dr. Atlee reports; "Prior to the introduction of Natural Childbirth resuscitation was a common problem in our department, and we were constantly suffering anxiety over babies that would not respond because they seemed doped. This anxiety has greatly disappeared among those of us who use the method, and it is very gratifying to have baby after baby cry immediately and lustily."

In Chapter 10 of his significant, if small, book on *Natural Childbirth,* Dr. Atlee says in summary: "We believe that the results we have obtained with both mother and baby justify *us* in continuing to employ this method. But if we can obtain such results with the meagre preparation and inadequate hospital facilities and services we are now providing, what might we not achieve if we could persuade more women to prepare for pregnancy and labor with the care that our young men prepare for war, and deliver them in hospitals architected and staffed to meet the end in view? Supposing also we could persuade ourselves as obstetricians to play a less active part in delivery and, wherever possible, allow the woman to feel that she is doing the job herself? Wouldn't the results be very much better, and the women in labor find a more satisfying experience than they do now?"

CONCLUSIONS

The recent extensions of preparation programs and rooming-in practices call for a revaluation of the hospital care of obstetrical patients. These newer practices emphasize, again, that, women who come to the hospital to have their babies are not sick, but well, people. For the soundest psychological reasons these hospital "patients" and those who visit them should not be exposed to hospital environments which relate to the care of the sick. In concept and function the hospital maternity unit should be complete in its own operation, ideally to be housed in a separate building and to include rooming-in facilities and class rooms. In the administration of such a unit it might be well to resurvey some of our routine hospital practices which seem to be tied up in knots called rules, and see how many are really applicable to a division serving so specific a function as maternity care.

The childbirth and parenthood experience, I believe, can be highly benefited by the type of preparation I have described provided it is judiciously administered. The fact that emotions can induce striking modifications in physiological function is no new thing but it does here bring to mind the words of Helen Heardman previously quoted, "How is it, that we have allowed women whose function is the reproduction of the race by muscular effort, to embark upon the heavy muscular effort of labour, without even a second of training—and in fear?"

FACTORS FOR SUCCESS

For success a preparation program must be a wholly cooperative effort on the part of all who share its responsibilities. The functions of doctors and nurses are especially interwoven and flourish best in an atmosphere which can be likened to the guild-spirit. An excellent way to foster such a spirit is the holding of regular interstaff conferences in which the work is reviewed, weak spots strengthened and objectives reemphasized.

Finally, the science of obstetrics must make use of all other sciences. Future developments are already being presaged by the increased emphasis on its psychological aspects. Those who direct research in obstetrics, as in other clinical sciences, ever must be aware of the irresistible tendency to select subjects for study because of the technical ease of their investigation. Many problems which now seem to lie beyond the present sphere and purview of science simply await methods of attack. These we must continue to seek. Tradition has its noble purposes but it also often encases inertia.

REFERENCES

1. Davis, C. D.: see ref. Chapter I.
2. Wiedenbach, E.: *Family Centered Maternity Nursing.* McGraw-Hill Book Co., New York, 1958.
3. Thoms, H.: *Understanding Natural Childbirth.* McGraw-Hill Book Co., New York, 1950.
4. Thoms, H.: The Preparation for Childbirth Program. The Obstetrical and Gynecological Survey, v. 10, 1955.
5. Thoms, H. and Karlovshy, E. D.: Two Thousand Deliveries under a Training for Childbirth Program. *Amer. J. Obstet. and Gynec.,* 61:205, 1951.
6. Atlee, H. B.: *Natural Childbirth.* Thomas, Springfield, 1956.

IV

PREPARATION FOR PARENTHOOD

ALMOST from the beginning of our experience we became aware that fathers as well as mothers were interested in learning about childbirth. Recognising this we instituted combined classes in the evening at a time when both could attend, usually from eight to ten. This became a large group with as many as 40 to 50 couples attending. In the question periods it soon became evident that many of these young people had interests adjunct to the baby's birth concerning the start of family life and their own roles in parenthood. We enlisted a pediatrician to talk about these aspects and on occasion had a psychiatrist talk about family life.

THE OPPORTUNITY TO LEARN

There is no question that many expectant parents wish to learn and talk about their future roles if given the chance. Talks on parenthood such as I envisage should be an elective, so to speak, and given early in pregnancy before the mothers' classes begin. The importance of giving them early has a number of advantages one being that the pregnancy itself often requires a considerable adjustment. Another is that these early weeks often are a "do nothing" period for many couples and is a time when they have more free time for learning together.

THE OBSTETRICIAN AND PARENTHOOD CLASSES

The obstetrician's interest in this aspect is natural enough. He is a doctor of health as well as disease and I hope the seeking of his advice in matters of everyday living has not been outmoded. Whether he will have the time and aptitude for devoting much time to this and other parts of the teaching program will be a matter for his decision. Certainly the words of Dr. F. A. Reynolds have much to say, *viz;*"[1] The demands of such care require an expenditure of physical and emotional energy on the part of the physician are quite impractical for the average obstetrician and could be made possible only by the limitation of practice to a relatively small number of patients." There can be no question that the obstetrician is in the key position in all preparation program activities and that his energy must be conserved. Few who have not been on the firing line know what it means to go short on sleep and rest for a week at a time and still be expected to give the utmost in judgement and skill to the patient in labor. Fortunately with such complete hospitalization for childbirth, additions to the obstetric team of specially trained nurses, nurse-midwives and other personnel can and must be made. We must see their valuable services in proper perspective and they must be given full recognition. It all takes doing but it can be done.

THE PEDIATRICIAN'S INTEREST

The desires of expectant parents to learn about their new roles is obviously related to pediatric practice. The extraordinary growth and success of the well baby conference in office and clinic practice has brought the pediatrician into intimate contact with parental problems as well as those of the child. We recognize the important part to be played by the pediatrician in our program by mothers being given the opportunity to talk with him. He is in a unique position to discuss with them such topics as breast feeding, rooming-in, the home coming and other subjects in parental-child relationships. But like the obstetrician his time too must be conserved. The social worker, the psychiatric nurse, the marriage counselor all have interests in parenthood preparation and their skills should be used. I know of one successful expectant parents' discussion group being carried on by a psychiatrically trained nurse, herself the mother of two, and no longer in active professional life. There must be others.

PREPARATION CLASSES

An adequate plan of instruction for parenthood preparation classes is something for experts yet to develop. However, with suggestions from varied sources I have taken it upon myself to outline four talks which might occupy the first part of a two hour discussion period. Question periods are of highest importance in this field for only through them may we learn something of the needs of these young people and something also of their thinking. As in the childbirth perparation classes previously described the first axiom here is to never underrate the intelligence of the group no matter how meager the educational background of some of its members appears to be. It is important also that the leaders of these classes be mature individuals and capable of stimulating discussion. I am strongly of the opinion that they should be adequately reimbursed for their effort. This not only preserves interest but insures repeating the course at regular intervals.

OUTLINE OF FOUR TALKS

The topics for discussion suggested for the four talks may be considered as jumping off places, details of development being left to leaders. An important thing to remember is that the talks are aimed at a wife and husband preparing *themselves* for parenthood and that specific child problems need not concern them at this time. Many of the topics suggested are discussed in other parts of the preparation program. Even so, I believe a specific program such as outlined here is useful and could be productive of good for its own future development.

TALK No. 1
Preparing for Parenthood

1. General considerations; outline of the course
2. Husband and wife can learn together
3. Reliance on the on-the-job experience
4. Children and marital happiness
5. Importance of a mutual desire for children
6. Acceptance of a boy or girl
7. The child's dependence and independence
8. Sacrifices and satisfactions of parents
9. Fathers and mothers in a complementary role
10. Imagined "intrusion" of a child in the marriage relationship
11. Effects of overindulgence and domination
12. The search for satisfaction; parents must grow too
13. What kind of love in marriage is desired?
14. Parenthood—a cohesive force
15. Economics of parenthood—family size
16. Importance of free discussion—in the classes, in the home
17. Sources for reading
18. The child as an individual

TALK No. 2
Heredity and Environment

1. Definitions
2. The science of genetics
3. Heredity characteristics
4. Heredity gives natural equipment
5. Acquired characteristics
6. Environment gives training, education, experience in society
7. Heredity principles: Mendel's law
8. Mendel and his experiments
9. Dominant and recessive influences
10. Determination of sex (x and y) chromosomes
11. Genes, the ultimate factors
12. Development of twins
13. Inheritance of physical and mental traits
14. Environment, the supreme challenge to parents
15. Importance of the home experience.
16. Marital tensions and children's maladjustments
17. Personality of child to be built around his intelligence.
18. Importance of early parental adjustments

TALK No. 3
The Newborn Baby

1. Helplessness at birth
2. Growth, the cardinal characteristic
3. Intrauterine activities of fetus
4. The reflexes at birth
5. Seeing and hearing
6. The nursing function
7. The rights of the child
8. Advantages of rooming-in
9. The child as an individual

TALK No. 4
Parenthood and Marriage

1. Adjustments for each in marriage
2. Interdependence in marriage—awareness of partnership
3. Immaturity in marriage—may cause resentment of pregnancy
4. Parenthood and the strengthening of marriage
5. Discipline in the home; self-discipline
6. The parents' right to pleasure
7. List of reading aids; Children's Bureau publications
8. Reading and discussing together
9. On-the-job experience to be depended on
10. Parents must accept their own capabilities and limitations
11. Exaggerated independence in marriage reflected in children
12. The mutual desire for success

In considering these topics and their timeliness as an introduction to pregnancy, so to speak, we might remind ourselves of the following;

(1) Most first pregnancies occur in the early months of marriages, a time when for each partner major adjustments are being made. And, this is true for *all* marriages. (2) The advent of pregnancy brings into marriage an entirely new aspect. It should and can be an important stabilizing influence. (3) If classes on parenthood preparation are kept on a broad basis free discussion

should be stimulated; important in the classroom, but more so in the home. (4) For most couples first pregnancies last a long, long, time and it is likely that subsequently they will never have so free an opportunity to learn together.

REFERENCES

1. Reynolds, P. A.: *Briefs.* Published by Maternity Center A., *19:* 14, 1955.

2. Thoms, H.: Implementation of a Preparation for Parenthood Program. *Obst. & Gyne.,* v. 2, p. 593, 1958.

V

SUPPORT DURING LABOR

THE role of the professional attendant to the woman in labor is well stated by Hattie Hemschemeyer, Associate Director of the Maternity Center Association of New York, who says;[1] The woman bearing a child is not ill, in most instances, but she is experiencing a supreme test of her role as a woman. Bearing children is not a fact to be achieved by training as an athlete trains; neither is it something that a physician, nurse or midwife can do for another human being. The role of all these is that of an assistant. To be effective in giving such assistance, the professional attendance must not only recognize the physical assets and liabilities of the individual and know how to deal with them but must understand the significance that deep family relationships have for the husband and wife."

In 1954, Ernestine Wiedenbach of the Yale School of Nursing, collaborated with me in writing an outline of labor support with a summary of results from the mother's viewpoint. This somewhat comprehensive study was one of the earliest publications on the subjects and it is not outmoded today. It is reprinted here almost in its entirety because of its present usefulness to those who like to know more about this aspect of Prepared Childbirth. Miss Wiedenbach is Associate Professor of Nursing at Yale and has had more experience in the teaching and practice of this subject in a university-sponsored program than anyone I know. Our paper follows;

SUPPORT DURING LABOR

Support during labor depends for its effectiveness not only on the sympathy and interest of those in attendance but on their comprehensive understanding of the physical and psychological aspects of the birth process and the details and importance of the preparation program. Effectiveness of support is also predicated on normal labor; that is, labor in a healthy woman in whom there is no cephalopelvic disproportion and no abnormal fetal position, in whom the soft parts are normally dilatable and the uterine contractions of proper regularity and of suitable force, and in whom delivery is possible without undue strain. A guiding principle is that expressed by Dr. Helene Deutsch, namely, "to find a technic of delivery in which the psychic value of the mother's active participation in the process is taken into account, and to reunite mother and child as soon as possible after birth."

Practices that we follow include the following. (1) We try to make the mother feel important as an individual. We think of her as the central figure in the situation. We include her in our conversations with others in attendance. We consult her when it is appropriate to do so, and we introduce ourselves and others who may enter her room. (2) We try to give her confidence in her environment. We keep her informed of her progress and condition. We stay with her, and, if we have to leave even for a brief time, we tell her why we are leaving and when to expect our return. We make sure that she is able to call for attendance (call light or buzzer) should she wish it. We tell her in advance of examinations or special procedures that may be carried out. We try to be gentle, considerate, and protective of her when carrying out such procedures. (3) We institute measures to promote relaxation. These measures include privacy (individual room); quiet surroundings; a cool cloth to forehead, if desired; back rub, if desired; a clean, dry pad under her, as necessary; and warmth—hot water bag, if desired. (4) We instruct her in techniques that lead to effective performance. These techniques are abdominal breathing, relaxation, pelvic rocking, pushing with expulsion contractions, and panting at the proper time. (5) We endeavor to encourage her at all times by voice, look, and manner, always speaking with sincerity and remembering that the eyes can smile as well as the lips and that actions in themselves often speak with profound impressiveness.

GENERAL OUTLINE

A general outline of the support procedures that we endeavor to carry out on all mothers, whether prepared or not, can be summarized in the following statement. In our management of labor, we try to carry out a definite pattern, following several principles. First, we keep the mother informed of her progress. She is told about the position of her baby and of its progress through the birth canal. The devious explanation, the hushed tone, or the overly sympathetic attitude are all studiously avoided. Second, the mother is in a private room and not left alone unless she desires it, which may be the case very early in labor when she is napping between contractions. In any event, an attendant (nurse, medical student, or physician) is immediately available. If the mother desires, she may have her husband with her until she is mived to the delivery room. The physician sees her at proper intervals, especially during certain important periods in the labor. Third, in prepared mothers, the techniques of relaxation and breathing are instituted when they are necessary. In unprepared mothers, an attempt is made to institute these techniques as far as possible. In the average labor, the time for this is usually when the external os is dilated about 4 cm. It is at about this time that the contractions are apt to be stronger and more regular. The relaxation position and abdominal breathing techniques can alleviate much of the woman's discomfort, which in turn will reinforce her confidence. If the husband is with his wife and has attended the classes for expectant parents, he knows something of what is going on. He is often helpful as a back rubber. This is done with the mother on her side in the general relaxation position and consists essentially of massage with firm pressure over the lower back. If at any time the mother's morale seems weakening, attention is immediately given. This attention may consist simply of encouragement, further instruction in relaxation, or the giving of a sedative. When the latter is given, the mother is told that it will help her relax, which it usually does.

THE CRITICAL PERIOD

The critical period of labor is at the end of the first stage when the cervix is almost fully dilated. This is the transition stage. It is at this time that the mother may show considerable anxiety and have more or less severe backache. Continuous attention and encouragement are important during this period. The mother is told that after 10 or 12 contractions she will experience relief. During this transition stage, sedation is often helpful or whiffs of gas may be given. Many women, however, pass through this period without too much discomfort, practicing relaxation during contractions and quietly dozing between times.

The relaxation and breathing techniques are also valuable in the second stage of labor. As each contraction finishes, the woman is instructed to take three or four breaths by abdominal breathing; this will assist her in continuing relaxation. She is told not to resist the expulsive effort of the uterus. She is kept informed as to the progress of the fetal head and is told that she will have a feeling of stretch during the actual delivery, also that soft panting breaths will prevent a too rapid delivery. Nitrous oxide or trichlorethylene (Trilene) is administered whenever the woman desires it, and infiltration anesthesia is used when episiotomy is done.

Most women who have been prepared and who have spontaneous births are quite aware of all that goes on during delivery, and immediately after this event they have a feeling of well-being and are inclined to be talkative. They are often quite interested in the expulsion of the placenta. Our practice is for the mother to remain in the delivery suite for at least one hour after the birth of her baby. The infant is usually put to the breast at some time during this period.

THE TRANSITION PERIOD

Experience has shown that in normal labor the period of greatest discomfort is almost universally atthe end of the first stage, the transition period. Soon after this, as the head begins to descend, the picture usually changes markedly, and the woman who may have been fussing about her discomfort settles down to the task before her. Anesthetic agents not only are not withheld during the second stage but are sometimes urged on the woman who is having too much discomfort but not asking for help. Those who are in attendance at this time should be wary of misinterpreting the facies of effort as that of pain.

Certain points need further emphasis. We are convinced that a woman's sense of security is enhanced by not being alone when she is in active labor, that she prefers to be in a private room, and that for most women the presence of the husband adds greatly to the sense of assurance and comfort.

During early labor the mother is permitted to move about, to sit or lie in bed as she desires. At any time during the first stage of labor, if she is having more discomfort than she is willing to bear, the physician sits with her for a while to find the cause of her difficulty. Something is done about it—encouragement, instruction, sedation, etc. Attendants must not expect that all women who have attended classes are equally well prepared or that they will go through an ideal birth experience. It must be impressed upon many women that the need for sedation to combat discomfort or to aid in relaxation does not in any sense represent failure on their part. The woman who is anxious to do well often sets too high a standard of accomplishment for herself and as a result may become discouraged when things do not proceed as rapidly or as satisfactorily as she fancied they would.

QUESTIONNAIRE

A questionnaire was used in order to obtain some evaluation of the mother's own assessment of her labor and delivery. It is usually filled out a day or two before the mother goes home and is of course voluntary on her part. The content is seen in the complete report of a 23-year-old primipara, formerly a stenographer. Her child was born in December, 1953.

1. Describe how you felt, what happened, what the contractions (pains) felt like, what you wanted to do or have done for you.
   (a) In the labor room.
"Between contractions I felt good. The contractions started with a slight pain, getting stronger, and then leaving. The nurse helped me do abdominal breathing when I thought I couldn't do it. I was not in the labor room too long until the contractions gave me a rather bearing down feeling."
   (b) In the delivery room before your baby's birth.
"I had a definite bearing down feeling with my contractions. I liked the idea of a mirror. I watched almost everything. I feel I had one of the best experiences I'll ever have in life."
   2. How did your labor start?
"The pains started as a small cramp, something like menstrual cramps."

3. What helped you during your labor and delivery?
"Abdominal breathing. Medicaments."

4. What did you mind during your labor and delivery?
No answer.

5. What were your first thoughts after the birth of your baby?
"I wanted to hold the baby. I was just relieved that it was all over."

(a) How did you feel?
"I felt just fine."

6. How did your delivery compare with what you expected?
"It was much easier than I expected and not so long as I expected."

7. If you have another baby, would you like to have it the same way as this one?
"Definitely."

8. Did you attend mothers' classes?
"Yes."

(a) What did you gain from the classes that helped you in your labor and delivery?
"I think the exercises helped me very much. Also the lectures we had in mother's classes gave me a clear picture of what would happen. That helped my mental attitude greatly. The tour of the hospital helped too. I knew exactly where I would go and what the equipment looked like. I believe the parent's classes helped, too."

9. We would value any suggestions you may have or any frank statement you would care to make that would help us in our guidance of mothers through childbirth.
No statement.

10. What is your impression of rooming-in?
"I think rooming-in is something all hospitals should have. There are many mothers with first babies who know nothing about caring for them. Rooming-in gives them a chance to learn how to take the best care of their babies. Also, a mother gets to know her baby before she goes home. Having the baby in the room with you helps pass the days quickly. My stay whizzed by. I would like to mention also that I received very good care during my stay."

RESULTS

Questionnaires similar to this one were received from 142 mothers; 83 of them had attended classes, and 59 had not. Of the mothers who attended classes, 29 were delivered by private physicians. Of those who did not, one was so delivered.

The group that did not attend is of particular interest for it is obvious from their answers that many of them have somewhat lower intellectual attainments than the majority of the women in the group that did attend classes. Their nonattendance at classes apparently was due to lack of interest. We recognize this as a challenge and suggest that a simpler and shorter form of class work may be desirable for such mothers. This would be aside from the regular program. The survey shows that of those who did attend (83), 76, or 92.7% of the mothers had a high school education. In the group that did not attend (59), 22, or 37.1%, had a high school education. In the group that attended classes, 79.5% of the mothers consulted a physician before the fifth month of pregnancy. Of those that did not attend, 30.5% said they consulted a physician before the fifth month; 15 did not answer.

In the group attending, the presence of the husband or relative was commented on in 77 instances in the 83 labors. It was emphasized as very helpful in 36 instances. In the group not attending, this was commented on in 47 instances in 59 labors and emphasized in 12 instances. One woman wrote, "So glad you love our husbands as much as we do"; this has its own message.

In answer to question 3, "What helped you during your labor and delivery?" 43 mothers who attended classes emphasized the confidence that was felt in the attention received, the presence of the husband, and the interest and helpfulness of the attendants. Thirty-seven mothers emphasized the help they received from practicing the relaxation and breathing techniques. Twenty-two mothers emphasized the aid received from the administration of medicaments. In the group not attending, 33 mothers emphasized the presence of the husband and help from attendants, five emphasized relaxation and breathing techniques, and 26 commented on medication. One woman stated tersely, "(1) Husband, (2) Demerol, (3) Nitrous oxide."

In response to question 4, "What did you mind during labor?" the answers that seem significant for us are as follows. Of the women who attended classes, seven minded episiotomy and stitches, four rectal examinations, 21 severe pain; two hypodermic injection, two noise, talking, etc. in delivery room, and one shaving with a dull razor. Of the women who did not attend, four minded episiotomy and stitches, four rectal examinations, 18 severe pain, and one noise, talking, etc. in delivery room. These expressions we believe, usually reflect some inattention or lack of skill on the part of attendants.

With regard to question 8, "What did you gain from classes that helped you in your labor delivery?" 58 of the mothers who attended emphasized the knowledge of physiology of childbirth. Fourteen mothers emphasized that the tour of the obstetric division gave familiarity of the labor and delivery rooms. Forty-six women emphasized the relaxation and breathing techniques. The importance of classes as a shared experience was also recorded. Certain short answers were meaningful. One woman wrote simply, "Peace of Mind," another, "What to expect and how to relax."

Twenty-eight women in both groups were further questioned as to their reaction to the rooming-in arrangement. There was no unfavorable comment, and all were enthusiastic in its favor. One woman finished a rather lengthy discussion on the subject with, "It is just nice to have the baby near you to look at, too."

COMMENT

We believe the results of the questionnaire have been helpful to us in evaluating our efforts in carrying out the program. We are convinced of the usefulness of planned and integrated support for all women during labor and urges its consideration as part of all labor and delivery room practice. Those attending parturient women can be more effectual in their ministrations if they are willing to adopt a definite labor support regimen, thoroughly understood as a cooperative enterprise. Greater benefits can come from such an endeavor if the experience of physicians and nurses is shared in regularly held conferences. The mother's point of view is often greatly helpful in pointing out weak spots in the program.

SUMMARY AND CONCLUSIONS

We believe that support in labor should provide an atmosphere of friendliness, interest, understanding, and encouragement coupled with effective comfort-producing measures that will enable the mother to put forth her best effort in the birth of her child. Everyone who attends her contributes to the effectiveness of such support. This includes her husband or other family member, physician, nurse, medical student, student nurse, porter, aid, etc. The more each participates wholeheartedly and cooperatively in giving support, the better will be the mother's experience.

REFERENCES

1. Hemschemeyer, H.: *American J. Nursing*, Jan., 1957.
2. Thoms, H. and Wiedenbach, E.: Support During Labor. *J. A. M. A.*, v. 156 p. 3, 1954.

VI

ROOMING-IN

Rooming-in is a hospital arrangement whereby a mother and her newborn are cared for in the same unit, where a two or four bassinet nursery is adjacent to the room in which the mother is housed, and where she can have the baby with her as much or as little as she desires and can see what is going on with her baby at any time. On the part of the mother's attendants rooming-in implies a special attitude of maternity care based on understanding some of the needs of the mother, the father and the infant in their interrelations. This physical arrangement is also advantageous in reducing the possibility of infection, especially nursery epidemics in the newborn. The specific over-all objective is to foster a natural and healthy start of family life.

Another advantage to rooming-in is promptness in attending the needs of the mother and infant especially in women who wish to breast-feed their child. The educational needs of the mother are greatly facilitated by rooming-in, in learning how to take care of her baby now and later and what changes to expect. This is true also of the father who becomes intimately acquainted with his newborn from the start and learns with the mother. Another value to the mother is found in her ability to share and compare experience with other mothers in the unit.

THE ROOMING-IN CONCEPT

In Ernestine Wiedenbach's book, Family Centered Maternity Nursing is this summary of the rooming-in concept.[1] "The atmosphere of the rooming-in unit is conducive to learning and is certainly homey, friendly, informal, permissive and relaxed. A mother is in it because she wants to be there. Although the baby's crib may be beside her bed and she has easy access to a supply of diapers, shirts, pads, etc., she is under no compulsion to care for her baby unless she wants to do so. The nurse will 'take over' or help her according to her wish or need. The mother may cuddle or hold her baby as she desires; but for an hour in the afternoon and again at night the baby is usually removed, in its crib, to the nearby nursery so that the mother may gain adequate rest. The mother is supported in her desire to feed her baby, whether it be by breast or bottle, and is helped with any aspect of her own or her baby's care. She has many opportunities to discuss her baby's program with her pediatrician. He may even examine it in her presence soon after its birth and again before the mother and baby go home. She is encouraged to ask questions freely and to discuss them with her doctor, with the nurse or with other mothers in the unit. Mealtimes are apt to be social occasions, especially when the unit has a dining table around which the mothers may gather. When the father comes to visit, he may, after washing his hands and putting on a clean gown, hold their baby, change it or feed it; or, if he prefers, he may watch the mother or the nurse care for it according to its needs."

A PERSONAL EXPERIENCE

Dr. Anne B. Cadwell,[2] a London physician in her published account of "Natural Childbirth at Yale—Diary of a Pregnancy" relates her experience as a mother in our clinic and writes under entry of January 19, 1953; "In the afternoon I moved down to rooming-in and the baby came in beside me which improved matters. There are two rooming-in units of four beds each. Each unit has its own little nursery and its own nurse. The babies stay beside the mother all the time, except during the afternoon rest and at night. After the milk is in, the babies are brought in to nurse whenever they seem hungry. During the day the mothers are taught how to look after their own babies, and to this end each baby has a box on the mother's bed-table containing clean shirts, nappies, blankets, cotton-wool, water for 'washing off' and a mild antiseptic for rinsing off hands. The bin for the ditties sits under the baby's crib so it is possible to give the baby all the attention it needs without moving from the bed. Any time the mother is tired, the nurse is always there to take over.

Visitors, (husbands and two others, one at a time) are allowed to hold the baby if they wish and put on a gown, and husbands are taught to care for the baby too. When I arrived in rooming-in I was given a chart to keep a record of the baby's activities during the day, number of feeds and time asleep and awake. The night nurses keep this at night. . . . It was nice to be able to see the baby, and at 9 p. m. she woke up having slept the 24 hours since she was born.

January 20 (2nd postpartum day): Today I went for a walk up the corridor with the nurse, and was up to the bath room. The baby slept all night and was hungry at 10 a. m., 3 p. m., and 10 p. m. She had about one ounce of glucose after each breast feed. I am interested to see how she regulates herself. As all the babies here get immediate attenion there is very little crying, although the babies in the general ward can be heard crying in the big nursery, where they are kept behind glass." (Dr. Cadwell was housed in one of our first two units adjacent to the general ward. The present units are far removed from the general nursery.)

In January, 1948, the first inclusive report of our rooming-in experience was published in *Pediatrics*[3]. This was entitled, "A Hospital Rooming-in Unit for Four Newborn Infants and Their Mothers." The authors were, Edith B. Jackson, M.D., Richard W. Olmstead, M.D., Alan Foord, M.D., Herbert Thoms, M.D., and Kate Hyder, R.N. I believe that this is the first extended report of a hospital effort of this kind, at least a university hospital. The premises set down here are unchanged today nor have the physical arrangements been significantly improved in our new floors designed for the purpose. Our conversion of a sun-porch in this first unit shows what can be done in a simple and efficient way without new bricks and mortar. The complete report appears here and may be repetitious to some extent. However, it is an historic document and does contain interesting information in many aspects of rooming-in.

INTRODUCTION

Rooming-in is the term currently in use to designate the hospital arrangement whereby a mother may have her newborn baby in a crib by her bedside whenever she wishes. The term was first used by Gesell and Ilg.[1] Such an arrangement was established for study purposes on the University Service of the Grace-New Haven Community Hospital in October 1946. The four-bed ward used for this purpose is known as the Rooming-In Unit. An account of development of this Unit with a few preliminary observations is the subject of this paper.

Because of the enthusiastic participation of fathers in the project from the day of its inception, the authors were inclined to entitle the paper, "Rooming-In for Parents and Newborns." The husband may be with his wife throughout the first stage of labor if mutually agreeable; under normal circumstances he may see his baby shortly after birth—even hold him; he may continue to get closely acquainted with his child day after day in the hospital, and watch his wife and the baby at nursing time if that happens to occur during visiting hours. This paternal participation has afforded obvious satisfaction to both parents which we believe is salutary for the baby. Indeed, the first major assumption in making plans for the Rooming-In Unit has been that a mother's satisfaction with herself and with the attention and care bestowed upon her (by husband, parents, members of medical and nursing staff) is the best guarantee for her inclination and ability to satisfy and comfort her baby;* the second major assumption has been that the infant's contentment not only bolsters the mother's self-confidence, but is the first requisite for his unimpeded growth and development (which includes his emotional development), for his uninhibited capacity to learn, and for his gradual acceptance of the disciplines and demands imposed by family and community life.

There are two main incentives for the revival of the rooming-in idea, representing respectively infantile and maternal needs. The first is the combined pediatric and psychiatric interest and inquiry concerning causative factors and possible preventive measures for the troublesome behavior disorders and neurotic manifestations of childhood. This inquiry has led in recent years to a critical re-evaluation of the procedures for infant care recommended during the past quarter century. Observations and study of disturbed children

---

* Compare statement of Middlemore:[2] "The experience of the mother as she tries to feed a fussy or inert baby will be as important as influence on him, albeit an indirect one, as anything he feels himself, for she cannot give him the breast comfortably unless she is herself at ease."

and parents have pointed to the hospital nursery regime for new-borns as one probable source of difficulty, with two chief trouble areas: (1) the separation of mother and infant after delivery, a frustrating experience for those mothers who want to love and enjoy their babies; (2) the imposition of a rigid schedule for both as a pattern of procedure from the time of the baby's birth throughout infancy with too little regard for newborn needs and gradual developmental changes, for individual variations or for the particular stresses of the mother in her adjustment to the care of the newborn child.[3, 8-19]

The other main incentive for the present interest in rooming-in comes from the joint psychologic and maternal protest against the harsh denial of parental privileges which the usual present day maternity ward procedures and hospital nursery care of newborns entail. It is probable that the mothers who have dared in recent years to protest are those who have found in the theory of dynamic psychology and in child-developmental data, support for their ardent wish for full enjoyment and mastery of the experience and responsibilities of motherhood.*

At the New Haven Hospital, for instance, the first mother to make a definite ante-natal request for permission to keep her baby in the same room with her after birth was convinced by her instinctive feelings, by her education in child analysis and by former experience with two babies born in Europe that rooming-together was the only right way for her. She wanted very much to nurse her baby on a flexible, ad lib schedule. The request, made in the summer of 1938, was supported by her husband, by her chosen pediatric adviser (both of whom were child analysts), and by her obstetrician; but it was denied as being contrary to the then accepted hospital procedure. As it happened, the mother's wish was unexpectedly gratified. At the time of the baby's birth she was admitted to an isolation ward because she had mumps and under

---

* It is noteworthy in this connection that Mrs. Frances P. Simsarian and Mrs. Roberta White, authors of an article entitled "Two Mothers Revolt"[4] in which they describe the pleasures and advantages of having the newborn baby beside them are listed in the Contributors' Column as a psychiatric social worker and a former teacher of psychology, respectively.

the demands for isolation technics it became advantageous for mother and newborn baby to be cared for in the same room.

Any direct and immediate follow-up of this first actual application of a rooming-in concept was impossible at that time for many different reasons. But there had already been started an indirect approach which led through pediatric channels to a somewhat sharper focus on the potential advantages of a close association for mothers and newborns. In 1937, under the authorization of Dr. Grover F. Powers, a three-month survey was undertaken of the problems for which mothers of newborns asked for help during the month after their discharge from the hospital. The evidence from even this brief survey indicated that the hospital care of mother and infant did not prepare the mother to understand her baby or to undertake its care with confidence. Mothers, especially of first-borns, were often afraid to handle the baby and often unnecessarily anxious about his normal reactions. They were not prepared for day-to-day changes, and often fell into difficulty trying to maintain the rigid schedule recommended by the "baby-doctor" at the hospital. The difficulty grew out of the disturbing conflict between their loyalty to the respected medical authority and their own observations and feelings. But perhaps the most important consideration highlighted by the survey was the fact that the pediatric interne rotating through the nursery was writing the discharge schedules and formulae for the babies with relatively little awareness of the variety of infantile and maternal reactions to the feeding situation and their possible importance for the future development of the baby. Having no clinical experience of family emotional problems with a new baby in the home, he seldom had an opportunity to see the result of his recommendations and was consequently seldom in the position of having to be seriously concerned with earliest everyday problems of mothers.

In order to offer clinic-status mothers a much needed pediatric supervision and at the same time to provide the pediatric internes with experience of newborn problems in the home, Dr. Powers instituted the home-visiting plan in the autumn of 1938.[5] According to this plan the pediatric interne working in the Nursery continued his supervision of the clinic-status newborn babies until they were six weeks of age and eligible for Well Baby Conference supervision.*

This home service taught the interne in a convincing way the variety of home, family and personality situations which the newborns entered on discharge from the hospital. It taught him not to expect a smooth accommodation of all the babies (and mothers) to a similar set schedule. He could accept the reasonableness of a flexible schedule in early infancy. Each interne had the opportunity to learn from his own experience the value of knowing the mothers and something about their home and family background for the understanding and management of the neonatal period both in the hospital and at home. He learned to temper the discharge orders with verbal encouragement to the mothers for changes according to individual situations.

The response of the mothers to such increased attention to their problems is important for our present considerations. They had, it seemed, been long afraid to bother the busy, scientific doctors with everyday matters of baby care. They had, accordingly, sought answers elsewhere for the little but challenging questions which kept coming up. However, once the doctors gave heed and valuable time, the suppressed eagerness of the mothers both to ask questions and to help in finding the right answers became manifest and merited further serious attention from the interne. For instance, a mother who was disappointed over the fact that the interne would be unable for technical reasons to make home visits with her to learn how to take care of him before she went home. Since senior members of the pediatric staff had been advocating a rooming-in plan, the interne had reason to be impressed by the mother's suggestion; and was glad to tell her that such an arrangement was under consideration. The mere mention of this incident in a professional article brought letters from two prospective mothers in distant cities asking for help and instruction in working out a rooming-in arrangement. This response lent further evidence to our point: that many parents, subservient to the supposed dictates of modern medicine, have suppressed their feelings about themselves

---

* Under auspices of City Health Department and Visiting Nurse Association of New Haven.

and their children as unworthy of scientific consideration, but have reached out eagerly for help wherever the slightest evidence of professional justification for their feelings has presented itself.

One of these two mothers seeking advice about a rooming-in arrangement wrote from Topeka, Kan., in December 1944. She and her husband, a psychiatrist, wanted a rooming-in arrangement to ensure an ad lib breastfeeding plan for their second child from the beginning, because they both felt that much of the difficulty with the first baby (then two years old) was referable to the baby's hospital experience with much screaming from hunger during the four-hour intervals. We replied with suggestions based on observations of the first rooming-in "experiments" on the maternity ward of our hospital in September and October 1944. The rooming-in plan was permitted them by the hospital authorities as an exceptional procedure (the husband was a member of the hospital staff) and, as the mother subsequently wrote, it worked out advantageously (February 1945).

The other mother writing from the environs of Boston made an even more ardent plea for help in effecting a rooming-in plan for her expected fourth child. With her first three children she "had resented keenly having my babies whisked away after nursing which resulted in my being depressed and restless and fuming to get out of the darn place and home as quickly as possible." In the ten-year interval between the birth of her third child and the present pregnancy she "did nursery school work and read, so that the knowledge of the needs of a baby are now added to my feelings." In this case, the mother's eager wish was not granted by the hospital authorities, but she has the satisfaction of knowing that her plea played a role in making it possible for other mothers elsewhere to have what she wanted for herself.

It was becoming more and more apparent that the pediatric, psychiatric and maternal considerations merged in the recognition of the potential value of a rooming-in arrangement for both mother and infant. It would certainly offer encouragement to mothers who wanted to nurse their babies by permitting a flexible ad lib feeding plan. Obstetric colleagues and nursing staff gave their cooperative interest to the first attempts of putting theory into practice as described in the following paragraphs.

The first rooming-in ventures on the maternity ward of our hospital took place in the fall of 1944, first with a primipara, then successively with two multiparae. The two latter, from underprivileged background and mothers of several children, greatly enjoyed the arrangement and each felt entirely comfortable and competent with a baby beside her, regardless of what anyone said. The primipara, on the other hand, although prepared for rooming-in prenatally and looking forward to it as a potential help in nursing her baby, was obviously sensitive to the apparent skepticism of some staff members to this first experiment of its kind on the ward. She developed a series of difficulties, had to give up nursing the baby and was unhappy.

Whereas the idea of rooming-in had been suggested to these first three mothers, the next three requested a rooming-in arrangement. Two were wives of members of the pediatric staff and the third was a psychiatric social worker in the Department of Pediatrics. Each was pregnant for the first time. They and their husbands were aware of the skepticism they would encounter, but none-the-less pressed for what they considered the advantages of rooming-in. In June, July and October, 1945, the three mothers in succession tried rooming-in on the maternity division of the private pavilion. In each case both the mother and the father very much enjoyed the closeness with the baby and they have remained strong advocates of the potential advantages of a rooming-together arrangement. However, the mothers felt uneasy or guilty in having to call a nurse for help every time it was needed, since the nurses on a busy service obviously found it difficult to answer unexpected demands at irregular times; but if the desired help was not promptly forthcoming, the mothers were uncomfortable.

This second series of "experiments" served chiefly to document the manifest interest of pediatric staff members in rooming-in and to emphasize its incompatibility under a single room arrangement with the regular hospital maternity service in the absence of additional nurses.

Dr. H. T., at the time Associate Professor in the Department of Obstetrics, sympathetic to the ideals of rooming-in, invited interdepartmental discussion of the subject in April 1946. At this time K. H., present in her newly accepted position as nursing supervisor in obstetrics, expressed active interest in trying to devise a workable plan for the nursing care of rooming-together mothers and babies.

During April and May 1946, a series of four more "experiments" was undertaken. A student nurse was assigned to "special" each mother-baby unit. They kept records of their nursing activities. As could be foreseen, the time required by the four different mothers varied considerably according to their personality needs. But even the average time expended in nursing care was not significantly in excess of that recommended for the combined nursing care of mother and baby according to the nursing care standards set up by the National Council of Nurses.

That, however, was not the crucial point; it was, rather, the fact that nursing coverage around the clock appeared essential for rooming-in mothers and babies on an ad lib schedule, especially for the first few days. This precluded, from the nursing administrative point of view, any possibility of offering adequate nursing care to the mother-infant combine in single rooms on the maternity service. K. H. recommended a four-bed rooming-in ward or unit as the practical solution.

The following essential facts permitted the adoption of a plan based on this recommendation in July, 1946, and the opening of the Rooming-In Unit for patients the end of October 1946:

(1) Representatives from the services directly involved with the hospital care of mothers and newborn infants were cordially in accord with the development of a rooming-in project.

(2) A little-used solarium on the maternity ward was assigned by the Department of Obstetrics for use as a Rooming-In Unit. This made it possible to increase rather than decrease the number of available maternity beds. Reconstruction of the solarium under the supervision of Dr. A. F., begun the end of September 1946, was completed in a month.

(3) Through the generosity of the Mead Johnson Company, Dr. Powers could offer fellowships for a pediatrician and for a nurse to assist in a rooming-in study.

(4) A nuclear group of one representative each from the Departments of Pediatrics and Obstetrics, from the Hospital Administration and from the Obstetric Nursing Service formed themselves into a policy-making committee for the development of both project and study plans.

The Rooming-In Policy Committee agreed that a unit with 24-

hour nursing coverage separate from the existing maternity division was essential to carrying out a satisfactory study of all aspects of the subject. The desire to provide nursing coverage at all times for the Rooming-In Unit was based on the following considerations:

(1) The constant presence of a nurse was felt to be of great importance to the peace of mind of the mothers.

(2) The entire project was in the nature of a study requiring close and constant observations on all activities within the Unit.

(3) The Unit was physically separated from the rest of the maternity division by doors and was on a separate signal system.

The continual nursing coverage was provided largely by student nurses under the direct supervision of the graduate nurse who was in charge of the Unit on a fellowship basis. The cooperation of the Yale School of Nursing made this plan possible.

DESCRIPTION OF THE ROOMING-IN UNIT AND EQUIPMENT

The solarium, a rectangular room 20′ x 38′ was reconstructed to provide a four-cubicle rooming-in ward with a partitioned-off section at the end of the room for use as a doctors' and nurses' office and contiguous nursery cubicles.

The ceiling and upper half of the two walls of the nursery and nurses' office are covered with sound absorbent material to soften usual hospital noise and sound of babies' crying. The acoustic treatment of the upper half of the two complete walls of the nursery and nurses' office is deemed particularly advisable because of the cubicle construction of the two sides within the room which for purposes of ventilation stop three feet short of the ceiling as does the cubicle construction between the mothers' beds. The upper half of all cubicle walls is clear glass; draw curtains for the glass are provided for privacy as desired. It is thus possible for adjacent and vis-a-vis mothers to see and converse with each other, and for any of the mothers to see into the nursery and nurses' office if they wish.

One of the most important considerations in constructing the Rooming-In Unit was that of making it as attractive and home-like as possible, in conformity with the ideal of comfort and ease in the treatment plan. The walls were painted pale rose color; the trim

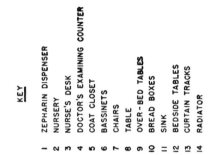

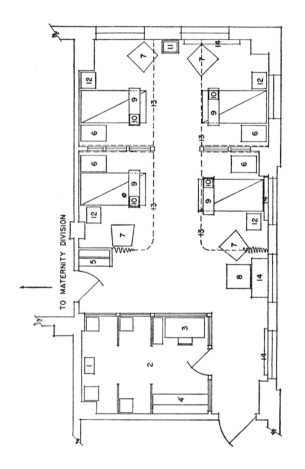

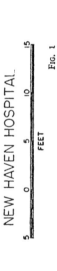

ROOMING-IN UNIT

NEW HAVEN HOSPITAL

FEET

Fig. 1

KEY

1   ZEPHARIN DISPENSER
2   NURSERY
3   NURSE'S DESK
4   DOCTOR'S EXAMINING COUNTER
5   COAT CLOSET
6   BASSINETS
7   CHAIRS
8   TABLE
9   OVER-BED TABLES
10 BREAD BOXES
11 SINK
12 BEDSIDE TABLES
13 CURTAIN TRACKS
14 RADIATOR

ivory. Chintz curtains were provided for all windows; monk's cloth curtains for use around the beds.

The equiptment provided for the Unit is the usual hospital type of bed, over-bed table, bedside stand and chair. Since the cost of installing a sink in the nursery was considered prohibitive, an alcohol dispenser for use with aqueous zephiran was substituted. The bassinets for the babies are of the usual type used in large nurseries, there being nothing on the market which offered advantages warranting purchase (several different types were tried out). A bread box with a drop-door in front is placed on each over-bed table to provide the mother with a protected storage place for supplies for the baby. In addition there are two rocking chairs and a table for the use of ambulatory mothers.

GENERAL PROCEDURES FOR ROOMING-IN PROJECT AND STUDY

I. Selection of mothers and preparatory interviews in Prenatal Clinic

In October 1946, two of us (E. B. J. and R. W. O.) started regular attendance at the Prenatal Clinic to select the mothers for the Rooming-In Unit. Since rooming-in could be offered to only four mothers at any one time, certain criteria of selection were necessarily established. Random choice was eliminated as a basis of selection, since it was considered psychologically unsound to impose a rooming-in arrangement on any mother unsympathetic to the idea. The following criteria were selected as the most applicable for the beginning of the project; they were aimed to include the mothers who would most profit from the arrangement, and to exclude those who would gain the least:

(1) The mother's wish to breastfeed her baby.

(2) The absence of gross emotional or social problems (obvious at time of interview).

(3) At least average intelligence of the mother (impression at time of interview).

(4) The mother's positive interest in rooming-in (including father's assent).

Parity has, to date, not been a criterion for selection. Actually the admixture of primiparous and multiparous mothers has, we believe, been an asset to the pleasant atmosphere of the Unit.

Changes in criteria will undoubtedly be indicated from time to time for study purposes. Even in the beginning, it has been difficult to adhere strictly to all four criteria. For instance, five mothers who knew during pregnancy that it was inadvisable for them to try to nurse were accepted as candidates, because they so strongly wanted rooming-in. The admixture of nursing and non-nursing mothers presents certain problems within the Unit, but the non-nursing mother apparently derives equal satisfaction from the facilities of rooming-in. We have also accepted several mothers with severe emotional difficulties which were not apparent in the first or second interviews. We felt in each case that the mother could be helped through rooming-in and that her exclusion would intensify the difficulty. We have, however, adhered strictly to the fourth criterion and never admitted a mother who did not want to have her baby with her.

The general plan has been to interview the mothers for the first time during the seventh or eighth month of pregnancy. (As the work has progressed we have tried to see the mothers earlier.) We introduced ourselves as the doctors who would later take care of their babies in the hospital. At the preliminary or screening interview, data were obtained in reference to the first three criteria only. No mention of rooming-in was ever made to the mother who did not want to nurse her baby, who was obviously disturbed or below par mentally. The intelligent, apparently well-adjusted mother who was eager to breastfeed her baby was interviewed again during a prenatal visit. At this second interview the pediatrician first encouraged the mothers' questions and then himself asked questions about the preparations she was making for the baby (Mothers' Classes, equipment, care of the breast, help in the home after the baby's birth, etc.) and her reasons for wanting to breastfeed. Only then was she asked, if she were given the choice between having her baby in the usual nursery arrangement or in a crib by her bedside, which she would prefer. Rooming-in was thus simply suggested as a theoretic alternative to the usual nursery arrangement with no attempt whatsoever to influence the mother's response.

If the mother expressed enthusiasm for the idea, she was told about the existence of the Rooming-In Unit. She was asked to talk over her interest with her husband and report to us again at her next prenatal visit. If at this time both she and her husband were enthusiastic, she was registered as a Rooming-In Candidate and was seen at subsequent visits in Prenatal Clinic. This may have been once or twice or several times, according to the length of time before delivery or the available time of the pediatrician. At each interview the pediatrician expressed his interest in the mother's well-being, in her interim questions and problems and he invited her spontaneous comments. He asked certain further questions about subjects already discussed, and also about her reading knowledge of maternal and infant care and about her hearsay knowledge of pregnancy and labor. He encouraged a discussion of her own reactions to pregnancy and about her anticipation of labor and child-birth, hoping both to gain information about the mother's concerns and to relieve her anxieties based on misapprehensions or unanswered questions. The mothers realized the dual purpose of the questions: to help them to a fuller preparation for the care and enjoyment of the child, and to gather data for study which might prove useful to other parents. In general they expressed appreciation for the interviews, thanking the doctor for his time. The more educated mothers added to their appreciation a voluntary statement of willingness to participate in any study that might be undertaken. The interviews were, of course, utilized by the pediatrician to orient the mothers to the Rooming-In Unit and its procedures and thereby to discuss various aspects of baby care with the mothers prenatally. It is hoped that time and personnel may sometime permit similar orienting interviews with the fathers before the baby is born.

Six weeks after the Rooming-In Unit was opened, a descriptive article about it appeared in a local newspaper. Prior to this publicity, the existence of the Unit was essentially unknown. During this period we were able to observe a succession of completely spontaneous responses to the suggestion of rooming-in. A majority of these mothers were smilingly enthusiastic, commenting variously, "If that were only possible!" "Gosh, I'd love that!" "Of course, after waiting so long, I would want to keep my baby with me!" The reasons given by those who preferred the usual hospital arrangement were most often that they would get less rest in the Rooming-In Unit, but also that it would not be so healthy for the babies, that the babies would be so spoiled if so much attention by the mothers, or that the mothers could not accept the limitation of visitors. In a few cases the mothers, themselves, preferred a rooming-in arrangement, but the husbands objected to it on the basis that their wives would not get enough rest.

As the existence of the Rooming-In Unit has become more generally known in the community (through the newspaper account, through recommendations of the Visiting Nurse Association in Mothers' Classes, and by direct referral of mothers who have enjoyed the Unit), an increasing number of mothers have spontaneously requested admission. Therefore, the details of procedures during preliminary interviews have had to vary somewhat to conform with the gradual changes in the situation. In addition to the mothers interviewed in the Prenatal Clinic, a few mothers under the care of private obstetricians have requested rooming-in. They have been interviewed and accepted on the same basis as mothers in the Prenatal Clinic.

During the first nine months of work (from October 1, 1946, to July 1, 1947) 434 mothers were interviewed. Their responses may be roughly classified as follows.

Rejected on basis of criteria 1, 2 and 3 199
　　(approximately two-thirds of these rejections were because the
　　mothers did not want to breastfeed)
Offered possibility of Rooming-In Arrangement 235
　　Wanted Rooming-In 175
　　Did not want Rooming-In 60

II. Procedures in the Unit

1. Admission of mothers to the Unit.

When a prospective rooming-in mother is admitted to the hospital in labor, the pediatrician and nurse on call for the Unit are notified and plans are made for her admission after delivery. There have been certain practical difficulties associated with the availability of only four beds. In order to justify constant nursing coverage of the Unit, we have attempted to keep the beds filled. Thus occasions have arisen when a mother, previously selected as a rooming-in candidate, delivers at a time when the Unit is filled and she must accordingly wait until a bed becomes available before she can be transferred to the Unit. On other occasions we have moved mothers who were not previously selected from the ward to the Unit in order to keep the Unit filled when no rooming-in mother was in labor. During the first eight months of operation, however, there have been only seven previously selected mothers who were unable to come into the Unit because of lack of space.

In the eight months from November 1, 1946, to July 1, 1947, there have been a total of 116 mothers in the Unit. 99 were admitted through Prenatal Clinic and 17 were under private obstetrical care. They were almost equally divided between primipara and multipara.

If a bed is available following delivery, mother and baby together are taken directly to the Unit. The father may accompany them and is allowed to remain for a short visit. After the father has left, the mother may keep the baby by her bedside, or if she prefers and particularly if the delivery has occurred at night, the baby may be taken to the Unit nursery. In this case he is returned to the mother's bedside whenever she requests or at the time of the first nursing.

As soon after the birth as possible the baby is examined by the pediatrician who then discusses the examination and the baby's condition with the mother. At this time, too, he helps to acquaint the mother with certain procedures in the Unit, and helps her with certain aspects of the care of the newborn baby.

2. Amount of time baby is at bedside.

During the course of her hospital stay, the mother is allowed to have the baby by her bedside as much of the time as she desires. During the first four nights it is generally suggested that the baby be removed to the nursery to insure the mother a restful night. Some mothers, however, have preferred to keep their babies by the bedside during this time and they have been allowed to do so. The period from 12:30 to 2:00 p. m. each day, just before the arrival of visitors, is usually a quiet rest period for the mothers, and many of them have preferred to have the baby in the Unit nursery at this time. It is impressed on each mother that the baby may be moved to the nursery or left by the bedside as she wishes. By the fifth day the majority of the mothers keep the babies beside them all the time. Except in occasional cases, a baby in the nursery is taken out to the mother for nursing when hungry.

3. Mother's care of the baby.

Throughout the mother's eight day hospitalization, an effort is made to give her the feeling that she need not assume any of the practical care of the baby, such as lifting him from the crib and diapering him. As she begins to feel energetic and expresses a desire to take care of the baby, she is allowed to do so. The nurse, in constant attendance, is ready at all times either to assume full care of the baby or to help and instruct, according to the mother's wish. During the first few days many mothers have had difficulty in lifting the babies from the bassinets onto their beds. The nurses make a special effort at these times to help them, to avoid any feeling of undue physical exertion on the mother's part. The bread box on the mother's over-bed table, containing the baby's supplies and the materials for the care of the mother's nipples and the cleaning of her hands, has proved an easy and satisfactory arrangement, probably more so than a self-contained bassinet unit, because the mothers can easily pull the over-bed table to the desired position. The mothers have been dextrous and uncomplaining in the handling of their babies while in bed. As already indicated, the reaction of the mothers toward assuming practical care of their babies has varied, some beginning almost at once to take complete care, while others, more hesitant, prefer to have the nurses do most of the care while they observe and learn. However, by the fourth or fifth day in the Unit, most of the mothers feel quite self-sufficient and confident and are caring for the babies entirely by themselves. Almost without exception, the mothers have spontaneously expressed at the time of discharge their feeling of confidence and their appreciation for the Unit facilities in making this possible.

4. Self-demand schedule for both mothers and infants.

The mothers have been encouraged to nurse their babies when they are awake and apparently hungry. Formulae are not routinely written but are ordered for any baby whose behavior indicates lack of satisfaction at the breast. Plain sterile water is available for the mothers to offer the babies who do not drop off to sleep easily after nursing. We shall not report here on the number and frequency of nursing periods under this regime other than to say that a definite peak in the number of nursing periods usually occurs on the four and fifth days, falling off again on the sixth and seventh days. Some mothers have become obviously fatigued during these peak days, and in these cases we have attempted to ease the mother's burden by providing occasional supplementary or complementary formulae, and by having the nurse feed the baby in the nursery so that the mother may rest or sleep. As far as possible the babies are weighed and their temperatures taken when they are awake to avoid waking them unnecessarily. Similarly, panning, bathing, etc., are provided for the mothers according to their need or readiness. The mothers have reacted favorably to this lack of absolute routine in hospital care, particularly the multiparous mothers, who have generally remembered unpleasantly the hospital interruption of sleep and rest during previous confinements.

5. Visiting in the Unit.

Because of the baby's presence by the mother's bedside, the number of visitors each mother may have has been limited to two other than her husband during the course of her hospital stay. There is an afternoon and an evening visiting hour; only one of the three visitors is allowed at any one time. (Occasional exceptions are made for out-of-town visitors.) This arrangement has diminished considerably the usual confusion at the time of hospital visiting hours and has, in general, met with the approval of the mothers. Obviously, visitors who have colds or any form of infection are excluded. Visitors may hold the baby (if awake); the father, in particular, is encouraged to do so. Before holding the baby, however, the visitor is required to wash his hands thoroughly and put on a gown. We have also encouraged the father's presence when the mother is nursing the baby. Almost all the fathers have shown a great interest in their babies. Many a one, who on the first day hesitated to hold the baby "for fear it would break," found it "a real thrill" subsequently, and confidently marched right in to the Unit, put on a gown, and expectantly waited for the baby to awake. Many of the fathers, too, have been interested in helping their wives get the baby in position for nursing, in giving the baby water or changing his diapers. This has proved a significant, practical help for the mothers in the first period of adjustment at home. Our observations have not indicated any disadvantages for the babies in allowing visitors to hold them. Specifically, no baby has had to be isolated for diarrhoea or skin infection.

6. Mothers' notes and Behavior Day Charts.

During the first three months of the project, the mothers were asked to keep notes about the babies' behavior and their own reactions. Sometimes these turned out to be merely notations of the clock time and the length of time spent in feeding and changing the baby. The notes, none-the-less, served the purpose of focusing the mother's attention on the details of the baby's reactions and day by day changes, and of reminding her of questions to ask doctor or nurse. Sometimes the notes described the baby's looks and actions and the mother's feelings in considerable detail. Almost every mother in the early weeks wrote notes about her pleasure of rooming-in. They often added constructive suggestions for improvement, some of which we were able to follow out. Hospital regulations for visitors have not permitted fulfillment of the unanimous wish of the multiparous mothers to see their other children and to have the children see them and the new baby; nor have the mothers been able to talk directly with the children by telephone until they are up and ambulatory.

In February, the use of Behavior Day Charts recommended by Dr. Arnold Gesell and Dr. Frances Ilg[1] was introduced to the mothers in the Unit. In general the mothers have been enthusiastic about filling in the chart and have wanted to continue it at home as illustration of the baby's progress. No pressure has been exerted on the few mothers who were disinclined or unable to keep a chart.

7. Nursing care .

The unified care of mother and baby has been a new and valued experience for all nurses working in the Unit. Each group of student nurses rotating through Rooming-In have volunteered statements of appreciation for the educational merits of the service and the opportunity "to do real nursing." The sincerity of this appreciation has been documented several times by requests from young married nurses who have had experience in the Unit to be registered as candidates for admission as soon as they have become pregnant.

GENERAL OBSERVATIONS AND TESTIMONIALS

The most frequent questions which skeptical colleagues have asked both before and after the Unit was opened are the following:

Won't it tire a mother to have her baby with her all the time?

Won't the mother be tired out having to listen to the crying of three other babies in addition to her own?

Wouldn't many mothers rather be alone in a room with a baby?

The multiparous mothers have generally stated that they preferred the rooming-in arrangement to the nursery regime and would certainly want it again in the event of another baby. They all wished they had had it with their first babies, and some were therefore inclined to feel that the limited bed space should be used principally for primiparous mothers. None of them felt that they got less rest in the Rooming-In Unit than during their previous confinements. Most of them stated positively that they actually felt more rested and peaceful under the rooming-in plan. One mother verbalized her comparative feelings thus: "It was like getting into a quiet country by-way after the glaring lights of Broadway!"

During the first three months we asked every mother how she reacted to the crying of her own baby and to that of the others. The answers were so uniform that we stopped asking as a regular procedure; but spontaneous comments in the same vein have continued to come. The multiparous mothers all referred to their previous worry in not knowing what was happening to the baby. Every time they heard crying from the nursery, each mother thought it might be her child and feared that nothing was being done about it. In the Rooming-In Unit, on the contrary, they found peace of mind in knowing what the baby was doing all the time. For both the multiparous and the primiparous mothers, crying is essentially a signal to them of the baby's normal response, which they are glad to hear. They do not pay attention to the crying of other babies (except on the few occasions when a baby's crying has been excessive) because they know the babies will get immediate attention. The acoustic-celotex serves its purpose of reducing the sharpness of the crying sound. However, it may be emphasized that because of the immediate attention given to crying babies, there is relatively little crying compared with that heard in a nursery. Visitors to the Unit have usually been surprised at the quietude.

According to our observations, the majority of mothers have definitely liked the four-bed arrangement. They have appreciated the opportunity of observing other mothers and babies, exchanging with each other the various comments of doctors and nurses, and in general talking among themselves about their mutual problems. Both the experienced and the inexperienced mothers have found it a valuable and enjoyable educational opportunity. Obviously the grouping which depends entirely on the hour and day of delivery has varied in the degree of congeniality. Only a very occasional mother, however, has shown inclination to keep to herself, apart from the general interest of the Unit. On a few occasions single rooms have been used for a mother and baby together, sometimes for the first two days postpartum and sometimes for the last two days of hospitalization. The mother's response to a single room arrangement is definitely more favorable to the later period.

A group of six university women from different parts of the country, who had been in the Rooming-In Unit at different times, were asked their opinion about the optimal arrangement for rooming-in. They definitely favored a four-bed unit with the possibility of partitioned or curtain privacy over a single private room or a double, semi-private room. These mothers had on their own initiative and on the basis of their own experience prepared a panel discussion about rooming-in to promote its educational values before a Child Study Group of graduate students' wives. This panel discussion was, indeed, the most gratifying spontaneous testimonial of our year's work. It was repeated, for the benefit of our several departments. As a result, participation of one or more mothers has been invited for professional discussion on the subject of rooming-in in our community.

SUMMARY AND CONCLUSIONS

Our report is limited to a discussion of the development of a Rooming-In Project in a teaching hospital, with a description of procedures and a few general current observations chiefly about parental responses. The over-all data from an eight-day Time Study has also been included in relation to procedures. Various aspects of the infantile welfare in relation to rooming-in, which have here received scant consideration, will form the basis of subsequent reports, as time and continued observation allow conclusions to take shape. In the meantime, we can merely restate a belief that the contentment and education which rooming-in does provide for certain parents is one safeguard for the normalcy of the development of the children of those parents. We are not holding a brief for rooming-in as a panacea. On the contrary, we believe there are many parents for whom it is not applicable; nor can it serve to prevent difficulties in children of very unhappy or disturbed parents. But we do believe that for the children of natural, happy and healthy parents, it can offer protection against some of the severe emotional difficulties of children which the routinized child care regimes of yesteryear have encouraged.

*References**

1. Gesell, A., Ilg, Frances L., Learned, Janet, and Ames, Louise B.: *Infant and Child in the Culture of Today,* Harper & Bros., New York, 1953.

2. Middlemore, Merell P.: *The Nursing Couple,* Hamish Hamilton Medical Books, London, 1944.

3. Moloney, J. C., Montgomery, J. C., and Trainham, Genevieve: The newborn, his family and the modern hospital, *Mod. Hosp.,* 67: 43, 1946.

4. Simsarian, F. P., and Taylor, R. W.: Two mothers revolt, *Child Study,* 22: 49, Winter, 1944-45.

5. Jackson, Edith B.: Prophylactic considerations for the neonatal period, *Am. J. of Orthopsychiat,* 15: 89, 1945.

6. McLendon, P. A., and Parks, J.: Nurseries designed for modern maternity, *Mod. Hosp.,* 65: 48, 1945.

7. Barnett, H. L.: Note on experiences with a rooming-in arrangement for newborn infants in a small hospital, *J. Pediat.,* 31: 49, 1947.

8. Aldrich, C. A., and Aldrich, Mary M.: *Babies are Human Beings,* The Macmillan Co., New York, 1941.

9. Aldrich, C. A.: Role of gratification in early development, *J. Pediat.,* 15: 578, 1938.

10. Bakwin, Ruth M., and Bakwin, H.: *Psychologic Care During Infancy and Childhood,* Appleton-Century Co., New York, 1942.

11. Department of Pediatrics of the Univ. of Chicago: Liberal infant feeding, *J. Am. Diet Assoc.,* 22: 602, 1946.

12. Gesell, A., and Ilg, Frances L.: *Feeding Behavior of Infants,* Lippincott Co., Philadelphia, 1937.

13. Jackson, Edith B.: Should mother and baby room together? *Am. J. Nursing, 46:* 17, 1946.

---

* These references were part of the original article.

14. Ribble, Margaret A.: *The Rights of Infants,* Columbia Univ. Press, New York, 1943.
15. Simsarian, F. P., and McLendon, P. A.: Feeding behavior of infant during first 12 weeks of life on a self-demand schedule, *J. Pediat., 20:* 93, 1942.
16. Simsarian, F. P., and McLendon, P. A.: Further records of self-demand schedule in infant feeding, *J. Pediat., 27:* 109, 1945.
17. Spock, B.: *The Common Sense Book of Baby and Child Care,* Duell, Sloan and Pearce, New York, 1946. (See also Pocket Book's edition.)
18. Trainham, G., Pilafian, G. J., and Kraft, R. M.: Case history of twins breast fed on self-demand regime, *J. Pediat., 27:* 97, 1945.
19. Trainham, G., and Montgomery, J. C.: Self-demand feeding for babies, *Am. J. Nursing, 46:* 767, 1946.

Here the report ends. Rooming-in no longer represents an innovation in maternity care for it is now available in some leading hospitals across the nation. As stated in the report, rooming-in is not for all mothers but experience has shown that most mothers who have been prepared do enjoy it and benefit by it.

Finally, rooming-in has important values for us other than those for parents and infants for it offers an unparalleled laboratory for research. Here, the words of J. H. Bradley[4] in *Patterns of Survival* come into important meaning; "It is odd that the nature of stars and the behavior of gases should have stimulated far more and abler inquiry than have the nature and behavior of man. To be sure, they are more gratifying subjects because they are more simple. But man can live without a knowledge of stars and gases, whereas he is finding it increasingly difficult to benefit from the vast and growing knowledge of everything else."

REFERENCES

1. Wiedenbach, E.: *Family-Centered Maternity Nursing.* Grune & Stratton, New York, 1958.
2. Cadwell, A. B.: Natural Childbirth at Yale—Diary of a Pregnancy. *The Medical Women's Federation Journal,* July, 1953.
3. Jackson E. *et al.:* A Hospital Rooming-in Unit for Four Newborn Infants and Their Mothers. *Pediatrics,* Jan., 1958. p. 28.
4. Bradley, J. H.: *Patterns of Survival.* Grune and Stratton, New York, 1952, p. 205.

VII

THE NURSE-MIDWIFE IN AMERICAN OBSTETRICS

Every year the obstetrical load in this country increases. In 1961, something like five million women are going to be delivered of babies and by 1970, six million is predicted. We should not only be concerned with safe hospital care for these women but with their satisfactions in the experience and the start of family life. It has been pointed out that the two areas which need the most attention in an inclusive hospital program are labor and delivery techniques and rooming-in procedures. One answer to more trained help in the former is found in the encouragement of the use of the nurse-midwife who is now functioning in some important teaching centers although in small numbers. She is ideally equipped to give and direct support during labor and also to conduct normal deliveries when called upon. In most European countries even in medical school hospitals well trained midwives deliver most of the women. In many places they are a part of the medical school teaching staff. That they are doing excellent work in Great Britain, Scandinavia and France has been attested by many American obstetricians who have surveyed their work.

NURSE-MIDWIVES FOR AMERICA

Just how helpful some women can be was voiced in 1931, by Professor B. P. Watson of Columbia University, who formerly taught at Edinburgh. Addressing an audience of American doctors he declared,[1] "A nurse can become just as expert and reliable in conducting a normal delivery, as a technician in doing a blood count or blood chemistry. . . . I should like to see every obstetrical hospital with a staff of trained midwives so that when the doctor sends in his patient he has the assurance that a normal delivery can be conducted in his absence."

Dr. Watson's words today are those of prophecy for the nurse-midwife in America is making a substantial beginning to come into her own as an important member of the hospital obstetric team. However, her numbers are still small, perhaps five hundred in the entire country and less than fifty being added each year. There are but four small schools for her training but already there are three universities who offer special programs for nurses who wish to become nurse-midwives. It is not generally realized that the nurse-midwife has been with us for over thirty years functioning usually as a teacher with local and state health boards. Today at Yale and a few other places she is an active participant in the work of the hospital obstetric staff, aiding in preparation classes, directing and giving labor support and teaching nurses.

AMERICAN COLLEGE OF NURSE-MIDWIFERY

In 1955, the American College of Nurse-midwifery came into being. Two years later the College became a member of the International Confederation of Midwives representing more than thirty countries throughout the world. Today, also, as stated above three of our leading universities are offering courses for midwife education and a number of leaders in obstetric thought have come to Dr. Watson's point of view. Dr. Arthur J. Lesser, Director of Health Services, U. S. Children's Bureau has this to say;[2] "With little prospect of being able to keep up with the increase in the number of births and with evidence of already deficiencies in maternity care, how will adequate care be provided by the end of this decade? The suggestion has been made by some prominent obstetricians that one contribution toward the solution of the problem lies in the increasing use of nurses who have had special training in midwifery to work in hospital obstetric departments. The acceptability of this suggestion for the United States will be tested during the next few years. It is only through study and demonstration that practice will become more responsive to the requirements of changing times."

EXPERIENCE AT JOHNS HOPKINS HOSPITAL

In 1958, Dr. N. J. Eastman of the Johns Hopkins Hospital, reported on the nurse-midwife program at that place, namely,[3] "I have now had experience with nurse-midwives in our Clinic in over 600 cases in which they have given complete maternity care to mothers under the supervision of the resident staff. In this entire experience, these young women have not made a single serious mistake, that is, a mistake which endangered the life of mother or child. . . . In the Prenatal Clinic, they take time to answer in detail the patient's puzzlements and in labor they never leave her. They are quick to spot the abnormal and quick to transfer such abnormalities to the obstetricians; and in the remaining perfectly normal cases they provide a type of maternity care which is superior."

Dr. C. Lee Buxton, now Director of the Yale Clinic in an address given in 1958, said,[4] "There are about 500 trained nurse-midwives in the country now, most of whom are members of the American College of Nurse-midwifery. I do not view, and I am sure nobody else has a right to view, a program to increase their numbers as infringing on the rights of obstetricians or in any way competing with obstetricians professionally or financially. . . . It seems essential to me that some such trained type of associate should be available to fulfill the needs of the future. We need this type of help, in fact, today and the future apparently holds in store for us an even more time-consuming preoccupation with details which can be supervised by the trained obstetrical specialist through the trained-nurse obstetrician."

A most practical suggestion comes from Sister Theophane Shoemaker, a graduate of the Maternity Center Association School for Nurse-midwives, now the Director of the Catholic Maternity Institute at Santa Fe, New Mexico. She recommends that every hospital with an obstetrical department could use at least four certified nurse-midwives, one for teaching parents, the other three to attend mothers in labor, one for each of the eight-hour work periods.

Another voice comes from Nova Scotia, that of H. B. Atlee, Professor of Obstetrics and Gynecology at Dalhousie University in Halifax. Earlier in his career Dr. Atlee served an internship in a London hospital where certified midwives are a part of the obstetrical staff. In a letter (1960) he writes, "Many, many times in the last thirty-five years here in Halifax, I have wished we had had a half-dozen such nurses in our hospital."

THE ROLE OF THE SPECIALIST

Dr. William F. Mengert is Professor of Obstetrics and Gynecology at the University of Illinois. In a presidential address given before the American Association of Obstetricians and Gynecologists (1958), he discussed future problems facing obstetrics in America. Here he states, "Obviously the specialist can only handle a small portion of the four million annual births in the United States. . . . There are some who advocate training of nurse-midwives, to act independently within the confines of the hospital while remaining under medical supervision. This may be the answer to a challenge of supplying proper obstetric care in an ever-expanding population. . . . The obstetrician who takes on an absurdly large number of patients frenetically to keep busy, to satisfy his ego, to make money or simply because his horizons do not encompass much more than the mechanics of birth must inevitably slough something. Obviously office obsterics, including patient contacts and teaching are the first to be discarded. We all know such male-midwives who virtually live in the hospital and appear at the office or home infrequently. True they work hard. I have known such men who delivered between 50 and 100 women each month throughout the year. Instead of sympathizing with the 'dear over-worked doctor,' I am appalled at the harm he does to obstetrics in general, through his failure to educate his own community regarding good maternity care. I don't believe that any physician can give adequate maternity care to more than 200 women a year. Multiply 200 by 10 or 12 prenatal office visits, by the number of hours required to attend each woman in labor and by the necessary puerperal care, and the truth of this statement becomes crystal clear."

No discussion of this subject should omit mentioning the pioneering efforts of the Maternity Center Association of New York and those of Dr. N. J. Eastman[3] at the Johns Hopkins Hospital. Both have shown conclusively that the nurse-midwife working in collaboration with the obstetrician can take excellent care of women throughout pregnancy, labor and the postpartum period. "As for the role which nurses with this training can play on the obstetric team, the transcendent contribution which they have to make is a unique personalized form of attention throughout pregnancy, labor and the puerperium. By training, temperament and outlook they are singularly fitted for this important mission."

NURSE-MIDWIVES IN A UNIVERSITY CLINIC

Dr. Eastman's convictions arise out of an experiment which was set up at the Johns Hopkins Hospital in 1953. This was to study the feasibility of training nurse-midwives in a university clinic, to evaluate the contributions they can make to maternity care and to ascertain the role which they might play on the obstetric team. The program was set up and carried through by nurse-midwives trained at the Maternity Center Association of New York. Nurses at the hospital who underwent training at their hands were referred to as Obstetric Assistants and under supervision by the medical staff they assumed complete responsibility for care throughout pregnancy and childbirth. In the prenatal period in addition to the routine examinations they gave each mother instructions in maternal changes and hygiene in pregnancy, growth and development of the baby, family relationships, diet, labor and delivery, and exercises in preparation for labor.

When the mother was in actual labor the Assistants remained with her, giving support, nursing care, and carrying out orders for medications and treatment within the limitations of the standing orders. The delivery of the baby and the responsibility of the mother and baby during the immediate postpartal period were also assumed by the Assistants. Medical consultation and supervision were always available. In the postpartal period the Assistant continued to assume responsibility under medical supervision, giving mothers instruction in postpartal exercises, care of the baby, and adjustment of the family to the new baby. Dr. Eastman says, "I have watched all this with my own eyes and am convinced that the meticulous type of care they give is the answer to the greatest weakness in American obstetrics, lack of emotional support both in pregnancy and labor."

NURSE-MIDWIVES AT YALE

My experience with nurse-midwives has not been quite as extensive as Dr. Eastman's but my opinion as to their worth on the hospital obstetric team is equally as enthusiastic. When we were setting up our Program in 1947, as I have mentioned, nurse-midwives who had been trained at the Maternity Center Association of New York joined in our effort. With us their chief function was that of preparing mothers, teaching nurses and giving support during labor. But, their usefulnes went much beyond these exercises for group after group of medical students requested instruction from them which was enthusiastically given and received.

Thus it is that I also have seen with my own eyes a good deal of what Dr. Eastman has reported and I will observe further that as a teacher of obstetrics I would rather have a medical student witness his first normal delivery under the management of an experienced nurse-midwife than under that of a verdant intern in the first part of his hospital training. I am confident that the student would be impressed with the skill and dignity which she would bring to the occasion.

The success of our experience with these able women may be judged by the fact that today at Yale not only do we have an expanded preparation program in which she has an important part but also in the Yale School of Nursing we have a program leading to certification in nurse-midwifery.

Ernestine Wiedenbach has discussed recently (1960) the opening opportunities for nurse midwifery in an article appearing in Nursing Outlook. "A cardinal principle in nurse-midwifery practice," she says, "is that it is carried on within the framework of medical care. This means that the nurse-midwives: will accept responsibility for care of only those expectant mothers who have been first examined by a medical practitioner of obstetrics and who have been designated by him as essentially normal, with expectation of normal, spontaneous delivery; will consult the medical practitioner of obstetrics and be guided by his recommendation should any complication or deviation from the normal present itself in the course of the mother's pregnancy or labor, including delivery; will make every effort to have the mother examined by the medical practitioner of obstetrics within one month of her expected confinement in order to double check the probability of the mother having a normal spontaneous delivery; and will arrange for the mother to have her final postpartum examination by the medical practitioner of obstetrics."

"It also means that the nurse-midwife will administer medications and carry out special treatment for mothers under her care only when sanctioned by standing or "stat" medical orders, and she has legal authority under some form of medical practice act to assume responsibility for management of a mother's labor—including conduct of her normal, spontaneous delivery. Under no circumstances does the nurse-midwife function as an independent practitioner in the United States. She functions either in association with a medical practitioner of obstetrics or on the staff of an agency whose medical and health practices relating to maternity care are supervised and controlled by a medical board or by specialists in obstetrics."

A report on nurse-midwifery training at the Columbia-Presbyterian Medical Center,[9] (April, 1961) tells of the graduate program in maternity nursing established there in 1955. Graduates receive a master of science degree from Columbia University and a certificate of nurse-midwifery from the Maternity Center Association who are associated with the project. In the Obstetric Service of the hospital, nurse-midwives deliver and care for mothers in normal pregnancy and delivery working with the resident physician who assumes full responsibility, writes all orders and is present in the delivery room.

TO CONCLUDE

I am confident that the nurse-midwife is beginning to function with ever widening usefulness in American obstetrics. The problems of the future primarily need more hands, doctors and nurses, and doctors have a duty to see to it not only to augment their own ranks with better trained doctors but with skillfully trained nurses and nurse-midwives. There must be established throughout the land better teaching facilities for both in our maternity hospitals. What Dr. Eastman says about the training, temperament and outlook of nurses in giving personal service and attention to the woman in pregnancy and labor is eminently true. She is particularly fitted to do so, and this has been true throughout the ages.

A celebrated midwife in the early Guilford group of colonists in Connecticut was Elizabeth Smithson. Her famous son-in-law, the cleric-physician Jared Eliot said of her in a funeral oration, "She knew when to exert herself vigorously and also when it was her strength to sit still."[9] This fine obstetric aphorism is expressive of qualities we can look for in the nurse-midwife as a part of the hospital obstetric team.

REFERENCES

1. Watson, B. P.: *Bull. New York Acad. Med.,* 6: 647, 1931.

2. Lesser, A. J.: *Briefs.* Pub. by Maternity Center Assn. of New York, Sept., 1960.

3. Eastman, N. J.: *Briefs,* v. 17, 8, 1953-54.

4. Buxton, C. L.: Changing Attitudes in American Obstetrics. *Bull. Maternal Welfare,* May-June, 1958.

5. Atlee, H. B.: (personal communication).

6. Mengert, W. F.: Obstetrics and Gynecology Today. Amer. J. Obstetrics and Gynecology. April, 1959.

7. Wiedenbach, E.: Quoted by *Briefs.* v. 24, no. 7, 1960.

8. The Stethoscope: Pub. by the Presbyterian Hospital v. XVI, no. 4, April, 1961.

9. Thoms, Herbert: *The Doctors Jared of Connecticut.* Hamden, 1958.

VIII

THE PROGRAM AND PRIVATE PRACTICE

T HE earliest contributions to the subject now embraced in Prepared Childbirth were made by physicians engaged in private practice. As far as I am aware the first adaptation of a program of this kind in a teaching clinic was made at Yale in 1946-47. In individualized private practice it is obvious that such a program will have individual patterns. Grantly Dick Read's methods of procedure are best outlined in his small volume called *The Birth of A Child* (1947) in which is found an account of this method of childbirth education, physical preparation and conduct of labor. He points out that much of the extra prenatal work in certain British clinics is done by the physiotherapist who in addition to teaching physical techniques may give elementary talks on pregnancy and labor. Dr. Dick Read deprecates the type of physician who is unwilling to give a proper amount of time to the patient in active labor. He points out that some aspects of the conduct of normal labor are sometimes neglected because the physician knows so little about it. "Normal labour" he writes, "is one of the most imperfectly understood of human functions because very few medical men have given the necessary time to study the full sequence of physiological events from beginning to end."

A PATIENT OF DR. READ'S

A first hand account of Dr. Dick Read's attendance at a labor comes to me from my niece who was his patient in 1950 at the birth of her first baby. In a letter from London shortly after the event she records, "When I was in early labor before Dr. Read came, there was a nurse there periodically who tried to tell me to relax and, most important to keep my eye on some fixed object in the room when the pain came and concentrate on it until the pain went. Dr. Read came in early, however, so all the rest of the instructions were from him. He did the usual, I suppose, of gentle rubbing on my lower spine when it ached terribly there, and just talking very quietly to relax me. When I got to the labor room I was in the second stage, of course, the pain was in front, and then it was Dr. Read who told me to concentrate on a fixed spot in the room during contractions and to hold my breath. Why this helps I don't know but it certainly seemed to. It was also he who told me when to bear down. Since his assistant was also there with Dr. Read a nurse was there a very little of the time. The nurse did only the necessary work of preparing the instruments, catheterizing me et cetera. Support all during labor was by Dr. Read but I believe that when he is not there the nurses know pretty well what to do. They seemed all to know what he wants with his patients and they try the relaxing business and spot fixing and holding of the breath too, I believe. As I remember, until things really began to happen toward the end, Dr. Read sat at my head, holding my hand, talking to me quietly some of the time and talking to his assistant, explaining what this sort of breathing meant, etc., which between contractions was even interesting to me. We joked and carried on quite a conversation at times, all of which helped a great deal I think. I suppose my case was a typical in some respects. Dr. Read was with me so much and I found this very reassuring indeed, but I also think that the next time it will not be necessary to have the physician with me so much and I believe, and hope, I can carry on by myself when it is necessary. And I also think the nurses can do what the physician has done, certainly in many technical ways, only they must have the quietness and understanding and easy-going way with them. They mustn't appear to be too professional and cool, at least with me."

AN AMERICAN PIONEER

An important pioneer in natural childbirth technics in this country is Dr. Blackwell Sawyer and his paper Experiences with the Labor Procedures of Grantly Dick Read, published in 1946 is a landmark. At a visit to the Yale Clinic in 1948, Dr. Sawyer told us about his experiences in private practice, of giving the exercises at office visits, etc. In his paper he says, "It would seem that the methods of Grantly Dick Read when carefully applied, is valuable in relieving the pain in normal childbirth in about nine out of ten women. The pain is relieved to a greater or less degree. Some women had no pain to speak of, to use their language, in the first stage, while others could not relax until Demerol was administered, after which the method succeeded. The effects during the second stage were very apparent, but the end of this stage required other help in some cases, that is, either ether anesthetic or novocain locally or both. . . . When the patient can afford it she has a special nurse. I stay in the hospital during labor, but at night I sleep there if labor is in progress. The nurse does not substitute for me in any way, but her main work is to prevent the patient being alone. The patient knows that I am in the obstetrical department of the hospital and that she is supposed to ask for me if she starts to feel panicky. This seldom happens. Usually the nurse will awaken me and ask me to look at the patient if she is getting tense—or if some change is coming, such as the end of the first stage. The patients say that the nurse is 'worth her weight in gold.' . . . The education of the woman's mind, in brief, is to teach her that at the end of her labor she is to meet her child for the first time. Every bit of emphasis I can bring to bear is focused on this—somewhat as Rockne used to key up his football teams for victory. With this in mind—and much can be said about it—the discomfort of childbirth becomes trivial to the woman."

FROM A GENERAL PRACTITIONER

Dr. Oliver Hayward has been a practitioner of general medicine in New Hampshire for 25 years. During this time he has lived with the change from frequent home deliveries to that of hospital deliveries for all. For the past 12 years he has been using prepared childbirth techniques in his obstetrical practice. A letter written in 1961 speaks of his experience; "After coming to New Hampshire I had a moderately busy obstetrical practice delivering from 12 to 20 cases a month and until the war at least half of them were delivered at home. I found that far and away the most important element in home deliveries was psychological. The patient was not sick and therefore going to the hospital, but was well and staying at home to have a baby. The presence of her husband, anxious to help and comforting in his understanding certainly relieved a great deal of tension which makes for pain. The presence of her children around the home was reassuring. She knew that they were not getting into trouble and she knew that she was not building up a big bill which the family could ill afford to pay. Another important point in home delivery was that the mechanics of the situation make it more difficult to interfere obstetrically. It is unwise and hasty obstetrical interference which causes an appreciable amount of the difficulty that I see."

"The problem is to translate the good things of home delivery to the hospital, i.e., with rooming-in and the presence of the husband in the labor and delivery rooms. The latter is completely impossible in a hospital where the nurses in charge have a horrified dread of this and believe that they could not stand the embarrassment of having a husband see the delivery of his wife. I have found that the tension which is apt to build up in the hospital can be markedly helped by prenatal instruction and exercises particularly in the case of the first baby. Another help which I use with success is to emphasize that childbirth is a normal and natural process and has been going on for a long time and that many aids are now available which make for more comfort and more efficiency in labor and delivery. I encourage the woman in labor to experiment for herself in what position works best, walking around or just standing and leaning over the bed, squatting, lying on her side, kneeling, etc. A large proportion of my patients today come to me already convinced that they want to use the techniques of natural childbirth and for these I encourage and put into practice the things which they are familiar with from their reading. I am able to devote considerable time to them and I find that as long as they have something to do and a way to do it their anxieties and therefore their pains are less. We have a nurse anesthetist whose very presence is reassuring and I have had her on my cases though usually giving no more than occasional whiffs of oxygen mixed with nitrous oxide for the pain of final cervical dilatation."

"I find that each case must be individualized, that the amount of help varies with the individual and with the circumstances. I think that mothers who go into labor with complete understanding on the part of their husbands and a knowledge of his pride in the event, do better. I therefore try to include the husband as far as possible in the prenatal instruction. We have tried at our hospital to have cheery surroundings and since we have a separate wing for obstetrics we try to make it seem less like a hospital and more like a place to go to have a healthy baby. We have been but partially successful in this because of the great emphasis on maintaining asepsis and therefore a lot of regulations about visitors. I am fortunate in my town in having a very well trained surgeon who has been trained obstetrically. If I get into trouble I call for him immediately and if I anticipate it I call before I am in it. His presence in the community has made the practice of obstetrics pleasant for me over the years."

"I suppose the cases who come to me are somewhat selected for those that do have already decided that they do not want the heavy sedation which others in the area use. I think I can say that in the last 25 years I have not delivered a patient under deep anesthesia or one who could not to a certain extent cooperate in the delivery. To this extent I suppose I am something of a man-midwife, but this does not bother me very much because I believe that the average patient deserves the right to choose such treatment and should not in any event be subjected to deep sedation or treated as a sick individual requiring strong medicine."

A NEW HAVEN OBSTETRICIAN

The following comments on the Prepared Childbirth Program are presented by a New Haven obstetrician associated with the Yale teaching staff but primarily engaged in private practice. "The class method of instruction is far superior to that of any individual instruction of my own. In the preparation for childbirth and the conduct of labor the patient gradually comes to realize that she is herself the prima donna of the pregnancy and not a patient upon whom the obstetrician practices his art, much as a surgeon removes an appendix. It is she who will have the baby with the assistance of her doctor and nurses. This is not a frightening prospect for a woman who is repeatedly assured that she can have relief whenever she wishes. Most patients get an emotional thrill from the experience and a feeling of dignity and accomplishment which they would never trade for unconsciousness or amnesia.

"I agree that support during labor is the most important factor. The assistance of the specially trained nurse here has been of inestimable value. This support requires more of the obstetrician's time but hours and minutes are not the true measure of wear and tear on the doctor. It is one thing to spend an hour in conversation with a sane, rational woman and quite another to listen to a shrieking maniac, even if she will remember nothing of it when she awakens next day. Second of importance, I would put the psychic preparation for labor and third the relaxing and breathing exercises. . . . For analgesic drugs, I usually use Demerol alone and a total dosage of 100 to 150 mg. suffices for the average case. It is given whenever the patient desires it. Novocain I use locally when episiotomy is done and repaired. I heartily agree with Dr. Read's observation that the transitional stage is the most uncomfortable part of labor, and that the patient feels much better when the bearing-down is established."

"Finally a word should be said about the babies. They are usually lively at birth and cry promptly and well. If the mother plans to nurse the infant it is usually put to breast within a half hour after birth and generally sucks vigorously. Also in summary I feel that the prepared childbirth program and the principles involved are of value in the conduct of any labor. For the woman who is physically and psychologically adaptable to the program no other technic for her delivery is as rewarding and as safe for her and her infant."

A NEW HAVEN PEDIATRICIAN

In discussing the prepared childbirth program and private practice it may be useful to hear from a pediatrician. Dr. Morris A. Wessel has written the following, "My association with the New Haven program began in 1948, when as a member of the pediatric resident staff, I was seeing expectant mothers in the Clinic at the 'prenatal pediatric interview.' At that time I was asked to meet with a group of expectant parents at the evening classes. Since entering the practice in 1951, I have continued to take part in these evening classes for expectant parents conducted by the University Obstetrical Service. I also see expectant fathers and mothers in my private office who have chosen me for their pediatrician. It has been satisfying to find that once it became known in the community that I preferred to see the expectant parents before the birth of their baby many of them have consulted me. Usually husband and wife come together in the latter months of the pregnancy period.

In the group sessions at the hospital and in the prenatal conferences at my office, questions asked fall into these categories; the health of the baby, equipment for the baby, care of the baby in the hospital and care of the baby after it comes home.

The rooming-in arrangement in which the mother and baby are brought together for most of the day provides an unusual setting for the doctor and nurse to be helpful. As I examine the newborn infant at the bedside, the mother as she watches often asks questions which are of concern to her; 'What about the shape of his head? Why are his eyelids so puffy? Are his feet all right, they look sort of crooked?' And, these questions go on to others. I am able right then and there to dispel any anxiety by assuring the mother of the normalcy of these things. Sometimes at first the mother handles her baby with a degree of awkwardness. She may find it difficult to put the baby to breast but the help of the nurse or doctor can readily show her how to arrange her position so that both she and the baby are comfortable. What a change one sees in the days that follow! Later as I watch the mother hold, diaper, feed and burp the baby it is likely that she will look up and say, 'I am so much more at ease than I was at first.' If it is visiting period I often see a father washing his hands, putting on a gown, and with a glint in his eye say, 'Now's my chance to change a diaper.' I can note also the relaxed manner in which they both now hold the baby."

"It is certain that these new parents have a sense of interest and concern for their baby which could never have happened so early under the conventional nursery system. Later, as the pediatrician of these parents I am aware of the specific concerns which they may have because of our prenatal talks together. With rooming-in it is a happy experience for the pediatrician to watch the new mother change in her capability to care for most of the infant's needs and while still in the hospital. I believe one of the strong features of the preparation is that it gives the pediatrician a fine opportunity to establish an early acquaintance with mothers and fathers. Parents and doctors can thus work together with better understanding from the start."

A CANADIAN COLLEAGUE

Dr. H. B. Atlee, the head of the department of Obstetrics and Gynecology at Dalhousie University in Halifax has been an exponent of prepared childbirth methods for a number of years. His recent book *The Gist of Obstetrics* is the most practical treatise on the conduct of pregnancy and labor written in our time. Everyone who attends women in childbirth can benefit from the wise words of this master obstetrician. Of prepared childbirth he writes, "Training for Natural Childbirth can be complicated or as simple as you care to make it, but the fundamental aim is to lead the woman into labor in as fearless and relaxed state of mind as possible. It is not a painless method of having a baby although a certain percentage go through with little pain but it is a method that 90 per cent of the women practicing it think sufficiently highly of to want to repeat with subsequent pregnancies."

Dr. Atlee speaks of the attitude of his clinic in these words, "We make a particular point of assuring these women that they are not irrevocably committed to the regime. If, at any time during labor, they find themselves so uncomfortable that they want a hypo they have only to ask for it. If they want an anesthetic at the end they only have to ask for it. What we find is that most primiparae have to have a single hypo of Demerol when the cervix is almost dilated. Some of the women ask for an anesthetic at the end. It should therefore not be claimed that it is painless."

Dr. Atlee's words about the effect of sedation and anesthesia on the baby deserve shouting from the housetops for it is in this area that we find the most striking benefit to be derived from such a program. "Then there is the matter of the baby," he writes, "While we have greatly lowered maternal mortality in pregnancy, the intranatal and neonatal death rate is still high. One of the commoner causes of mortality seems to be asphyxia in one form or another. If we dope the mother heavily during labor and wind up by putting her under what is to all intents and purposes surgical anesthesia her baby is born doped and does not respond well to the stimulus of life. Every minute that proper breathing is delayed means damage to brain cells, and since there appear to be enough dimwits about, it would seem we might serve a useful purpose by trying to lessen their numbers. Most women properly conditioned are able to go through labor either without a sedative, or with a single hypodermic when the cervix is almost fully dilated, with a local anesthesia for the episiotomy at the end, and are fully conscious when the baby is born. As a result the baby cries lustily and at once."

Dr. Atlee's forthright statements reveal often the depth and devotion of his spirit. Nowhere is this seen better than in his words "To Men of Conscience." They belong in every textbook of obstetrics. He writes, "You will hear of those who either directly order, or have private understandings with nurses, to hold back delivery when they are delayed in reaching the Case Room. This is usually accomplished by pushing the woman rapidly and deeply under general anesthesia, and holding her legs together and pressing them down on the table. Babies have been killed or become serious problems in the resuscitation, though this nefarious and dangerous practice. Our prime interest in obstetrics should be to get a live, undamaged baby, and not to arrange matters so that we can sleep a little longer before going to our patient's aid. A baby is more likely to live and be undamaged if it is born when it should be born, even if we are not present, than if held back by force or anesthesia until we deign to appear on the scene. IN THE NAME OF THE UNBORN, I BEG YOU TO LISTEN TO THE STILL SMALL VOICE IN THIS MATTER,"

A GENERAL PRACTITIONER

A general practitioner in rural Connecticut writes of his experience, "All deliveries were conducted at a general hospital. The nurses and resident staff were not trained in the methods of natural childbirth, nor in the supportive measures so necessary in the successful carrying out of this procedure. The delivery suite is so arranged that the labor rooms are next to the delivery rooms and two patients were usually in the same labor room. This created a most difficult problem in the manner of support during labor as frequently the patient attemping natural childbirth was exposed to the agonizing and terrifying cries of the uninitiated mother in labor and to sounds coming from the delivery room during a delivery. This environment had a bad effect as several mothers told me that they could feel themselves getting tensed and that they could feel that their contractions were becoming pains after a prolonged exposure to another mother who was not attemping natural childbirth. . . .

"It would seem that natural childbirth need not be limited to only those in teaching centers where the best of facilities are available for the fuller use and development of the techniques of natural childbirth. Any physician doing obstetrics has within his grasp the necessary knowledge whereby with a little interest he can offer the expectant mother an experience in having a baby that will be most satisfying to her and is frequently distinctly pleasurable. These patients who have experienced natural childbirth are very grateful patients and are the biggest boosters of the method. Their enthusiasm is spreading and it is understandable that more and more mothers are desirous of having their babies this easier and more satisfying way. The physician doing obstetrics should lead the way."

A NEW HAVEN OBSTETRICIAN

At my request, a New Haven obstetrician who has been using prepared childbirth in his practice since its inauguration, has submitted the following statement, (1961). "The progressive development of natural childbirth techniques in American obstetrics has been held back to some extent not only by an excess of zeal and missionary spirit on the part of some of its proponents, but also by the intolerant attitude of some of the opponents. Properly used prepared childbirth offers a method of obstetrical care which is far superior for certain patients than any other method known to me and it has enriched our understanding of the management of *all* obstetrical patients. Some patients find this type of delivery a most exciting and gratifying experience which they remember with pleasure for many years and count among the most rewarding experiences of a lifetime. Surely such patients should not be deprived of the psychological benefits of such an experience particularly when there is a bonus of added safety for both mother and child.

"The question may be raised; who are these patients and how does one identify them and prepare them for this kind of childbirth? In practice I find that I can make an intelligent guess but no precise prognosis as to how a patient will react to labor when the time comes. The greatest enthusiasm for natural childbirth is found among young, healthy, intelligent women with wanted pregnancies. In this area the wives of university students and resident-staff physicians are almost invariably in this group. Sometimes the height of enthusiasm develops during the course of labor in the most unpromising material, particularly if the labor is unexpectedly comfortable and rapid." "I prefer all patients to be prepared for this type of childbirth since they seem to benefit from the preparation regardless of how they are eventually delivered. Therefore, my patients are sent to the hospital classes for instruction and familiarization with the facilities for labor, delivery and rooming-in. Office visits furnish further indoctrination directed particularly to the prevention of over-anxiety or panic in labor. This is aided by establishing confidence and good rapport.

"No patient is ever promised a specific type of anesthesia or delivery, and indeed, it is repeatedly emphasized that the conduct of labor and delivery are determined by the obstetrical requirements, the patient's comfort and her own desire for anesthesia. These things can only be evaluated during labor. It is also emphasized that the pain of labor can be relieved satisfactorily one way or another and that any time the patient feels the need for relief something will be done for her. The acceptance of such assurrances is essential since without it patients often ask for medication long before they really need it. A well-supported patient in an individual labor room will usually go through labor comfortably on surprisingly little medication one or more doses of Demerol 50-75 mg. usually sufficing for the first stage. Nitrous oxide with contractions only is usually given during the transition and second stage and xylocaine used for the episiotomy and repair. If labor can be conducted comfortably in this way the patient is awake and lucid throughout and able to assist actively in the delivery of the baby. This kind of delivery is what prepared childbirth means to me. It is to be noted that its essence is not the withholding of anesthesia, but rather the use of other means to reduce the need for anesthesia. With proper preparation and good support in labor I find that I am now delivering a majority of my patients in this way.

"One opponent of this approach to childbirth has suggested that if you scratch the surface of a woman who enjoys the natural childbirth you will find a psychopathic personality. This is certainly not true in my experience. One does occasionally see a determinded woman, accustomed to ordering her own affairs who resents the use of anesthesia and a forceps delivery because she hates to yield her place on the driver's seat. Even so, with these patients I question whether it is good therapy to seize upon the occasion of delivery as a suitable time to argue against her wishes in these matters.

"In my experience the great majority of prepared childbirth patients are exceptionally well adjusted women and the elation and satisfaction which they experience must be seen to be appreciated. I cannot regard them as pathological considering some of the lesser accomplishments that women become elated about."

A BOSTON OBSTETRICIAN

One of the leading specialists in Boston who observed the Yale Program in its early years and subsequently adopted much of its philosophy in his own practice, writes of present conditions here, (1961). His letter is highly significant for heavy sedation in obstetrics has long been popular in that area and a great deal of research on the subject has been published from teaching hospitals there. He writes,

"At the present time there is no formal training for Natural Childbirth in any of the teaching hospitals in Boston. There are, however, a few nurse instructors who conduct private classes for interested patients for a moderate fee.

"During the past ten years there has unquestionably been a great lessening in the hostility of the qualified obstetricians in this community toward Natural Childbirth and an increasing tolerance if not enthusiasm for the method. Many are now willing to allow a patient to carry through labor and delivery without medication or anesthesia if she strongly desires to do so and an increasing number are willing to try to make the experience a rewarding one for the mother. The frequent presence on private services and patients who have been fully conscious and cooperative in labor has had a subtle effect on the professional staff, nursing and medical alike. It is evident that there is more consideration for the patient and a gentler attitude on the labor floor and in the recovery areas than was true in the day when every patient was comatose or thrashing about in wild excitement from heavy medication.

"In most of the hospitals in the metropolitan area of Boston, the physical arrangements and the administrative policies are such that if the obstetrician so desires, patients who are not heavily medicated may remain in their own rooms during labor and the husbands may be present until the patients move to the delivery room. To the best of my knowledge the presence of the husband in the delivery room itself is not permitted in any of the urban hospitals.

"In my own practice as the years have gone by, I have found a steady drop in the number of patients who request oblivion in labor; in fact, I now find myself mildly surprised when anyone does ask to be completely knocked out. The majority of my patients are alert and conscious through labor and delivery and I believe thoroughly enjoy it.

"I tend to avoid the term 'Natural Childbirth' as it has different connotations for one person and another. My belief is that labor and delivery should be a pleasant experience for the mother. For most women pain is not unbearable and can be minimized by judicious use of drugs like Nisentil or Demerol during labor and local anesthesia, pudenal block or even saddle block or epidural anesthesia at delivery. A positive and encouraging attitude on the part of the physician and confidence in his skill and interest on the part of the patient do much to reduce the need for medication. It seems to me that the patient's confidence may be achieved by personal rapport with her obstetrician or from formal classes. In many instances it is of little importance how this is achieved. In the occasional instance, however, I feel that those who have been too thoroughly indoctrinated in the lore of 'Natural Childbirth' may suffer. Such patients are extremely reluctant to accept the help of medication or any form of anesthesia even though pain is severe. If these individuals finally accept help they often carry away a feeling of failure and if they hold out to the bitter end, some retain a deep fear or dread of another labor.

"There is, I feel, less danger of this if the obstetrician has emphasized from the beginning the fact that there is no disgrace in accepting as much or as little help during labor as is necessary to make the experience a pleasant one. In other words, it is necessary to make it very clear to some patients that labor should be a happy and rewarding experience and not a test of endurance.

"As the years go by, I find that I tend to deviate more and more from the orthodox training for Natural Childbirth and make greater use of my own knowledge of the individual patient's capability and attitude and tendency to rely on me. Unquestionably this makes easier the management of labor when variations from the normal course occur. . . .

"In conclusion, then, I think it is fair to say the majority of patients may safely go through labor and delivery alert and cooperative and that the experience may be a happy one provided the obstetrician is willing to spend a little extra time in explaining and teaching during the prenatal course and provided also that he is willing personally to supervise the course of labor and give adequate support and encouragement at this time."

IX

THE CHALLENGE IN AMERICAN OBSTETRICS

AN editorial in the *Ladies Home Journal* (April, 1960) entitled "Doctors Can't Do It Alone," shows a deep understanding about many of the things written about in this book. At the start it poses this question;[1] "Is the mere fact of survival all there is to this business of maternity care? When we discharge from the hospital a living mother with physical and mental scars from a highly dramatic experience, and a child living but brain damaged because no one was around to recognise early signs of the *baby-in-utero* being in distress, is that job well done? So asked a distinguished physician, on the obstetrical staff of one of the greatest teaching hospitals in the world, of a professional gathering. His remarks were typical of some note of self-criticism which is spreading throughout the obstetrical profession today."

ASSEMBLY-LINE METHODS

This editorial also quoted this statement from a publication of the U. S. Childrens' Bureau which reads; "The most prevalent criticism . . . (leveled) at maternity care is our assembly-line methods of managing patients, especially the fact that they are often left alone throughout most of the labor . . . There can be no question about the validity of this criticism." And, according to the editorial; "Obstetrical leadership is admitting with greater and greater candor that it has become physically impossible for most doctors to be in attendance during the long hours of labor. The director of obstetrics of a great medical school told a medical congress that most obstetrics in this country is what he called 'perineal obstetrics.' This he described as the arrival of the obstetrician at about the time the baby's head first shows as the mother is

91

being taken to the delivery room. . . . Almost every doctor who delivers babies in anything smaller than a large metropolitan hospital will admit in private that he relies until he gets there on the experience and common sense of the nurses on duty in the labor room. Often he relies on the nurses to tell him *when* to get there."

Speaking of the nurse-midwife the authors say, "Most Americans are unaware that trained midwives, working under medical direction are commonplace in every western except our own and Canada; these women perform many of the duties surrounding childbirth that our own physicians hold only themselves responsible for. These duties include prenatal examinations, psychological support, and constant expert care during labor. In many countries midwives actually conduct normal deliveries. There is already a nucleus of such women in the United States, calling themselves nurse-midwives. The high standards already set for them include a nursing degree, postgraduate experience and as much as a year and a half of theoretical and clinical experience in obstetrics."

THE SPREADING TIDE

The challenge which confronts American Obstetrics involves raising its sights in developing all aspects of childbirth to a degree consistent with their importance in our culture. That this is happening to a considerable degree is witnessed by the number of programs now going on throughout the nation. An idea of what is going on in the New York area can be gained from an article appearing in the *New York Times* of January 28, 1961. This pointed out that couples expecting their first child can turn to many sources for help and information in addition to that given by their doctor. Many New York hospitals offer prenatal courses without charge. Most of them, however, offer the courses only to prospective parents who have registered with them for the delivery of their baby.

Prenatal or expectant parents courses usually go beyond the actual birth of the baby. They offer instructions on baby care, layette lists, formula making and suggested reading lists. During the classes life-size dolls are used for diapering and other practice. Films on birth and family life, group discussions and lectures by trained nurses and other professionals in the baby-care field round out the classes.

At Mount Sinai Hospital for example, education for childbirth courses are given free to prospective mothers registered at the hospital. Afternoon sessions for the mothers-to-be, or evening sessions for both parents-to-be, are given once a week for seven weeks.

At Flower and Fifth Avenue Hospitals a woman who is registered for delivery of her baby is offered a prenatal course for $15. This same course is open for other parents-to-be for $25.

In addition to hospitals, other sources that offer courses include Visiting Nurse Service of New York, the Maternity Center Association and the American Red Cross. The latter offers free expectant-parent classes. They are held in the local chapter head-quarters. However, most of the chapters have now full classes. According to a spokesman no new applicants can be enrolled for the next two months."

OTHER PROGRAMS

There are reports of other programs from other parts of the country. From the far west we learn of much activity and in some areas monthly bulletins are sent to enrollees and "graduates" of programs. A recent report from Seattle tells of 12 out of 20 hospitals which have some form of rooming-in, three have regular classes for expectant parents, 17 allow husbands to be with their wives during labor. Classes for mothers are also found in Seattle at the Visiting Nurse Association, the Red Cross and the Y.W.C.A. This information comes from a Newsletter of the Seattle Association for Childbirth Education. (October, 1960).

EVENTS IN ENGLAND

What has taken place in England since the death of the two important pioneers, Grantly Dick Read and Helen Heardman was foreshadowed in letters received by me, one from a friend of Mrs. Heardman and the other from Dr. Dick Read a year before his death. Miss K. D. Francis writing from the Royal National Orthopaedic Hospital, London, (October 8, 1949) says,[2] "I think the fact that during the past two years two London teaching hospitals have incorporated her methods, (Mrs. Heardman's), in addition to Leeds and Manchester in the provinces proves her work will go on in England as well as America."

A letter from Grantly Dick Read (August 8, 1957), is also revelatory of changes in Britain and tells us something of the writer at the time of his retirement from clinical practice. Speaking of the term, "Natural Childbirth," he writes,[3] "The name hasn't altogether found favour because it was adopted after my first little book in 1933 and remained very largely for the name of the system, whereas one could naturally have seen that the simplicity of it was self-condemning. It was never meant to be a descriptive term any more than Smith describes all the Smiths. Consequently it is called all sorts of things very largely by those who want to claim some initiating influence in this work."

About the introduction of nurse-midwives into American obstetrics Dr. Dick Read comments, "I did get hold of the *American Journal of Obstetrics and Gynecology* and read an article on midwives for America, which made me laugh a lot. Do you happen to remember by any chance the ribaldry that met my suggestion that midwives would be a great asset to American gynecologists when I was in America in 1947? . . . So times have changed, haven't they. Times have changed in many, many ways, because now, considerably influenced by your work at the Grace-New Haven Hospital the natural childbirth methods have definitely made a very big impression on America. . . . But on the whole I find nothing new whatever has been added to the original teaching except the environmental variations necessary to provide for the wishes and desires of the patients. . . . For my own part I have retired, and although I have not left the lists, I am not a practicing member any longer. . . . But things are getting better and antenatal classes have been started now and in most of the public health centres and many of the big hospitals there are also classes but they are still searching for a name because it would be difficult for them to suffer from a change of face after twenty-five years."

I am confident that Grantly Dick Read will be remembered as an obstetrician who made a lifetime pursuit of an idea which is becoming fundamental in modern obstetrics, namely, that with proper preliminary training and skillful attendance most women can go through childbirth with a minimum of discomfort and with a heightened sense of satisfaction. At the time of his death I wrote an appreciation of him and his work for the Journal of the History of Medicine. I was gratified later to see that my words received reprinting in his own country. A final paragraph reads;[4] "In his own country Read became a controversial figure chiefly because of his disbelief in the existing order of obstetrical procedure and his outspoken expression against those who did not share his views. In letters to friends in this country he always expressed his deep disappointment in the slowness of what he considered obstetrical progress to be. However, in later years he had the satisfaction of seeing that much of his basic thinking about the psychology of childbirth was gaining wide acceptance. From present evidence in American texts it is likely that his name will be regarded as one of historic significance for a long time to come."

FAMILY CENTERED MATERNITY CARE

The challenge that faces American obstetrics today I hope is expressed in the closing words of my recent book *Our Obstetric Heritage.*[5]

"The broad aspects of these new programs involve preparation not only for the birth process but for the start of family life. Today, more than ever the responsibilities of parents are receiving wide attention. Child-parent relationships even in earliest contacts are said to have potentialities for good or evil little suspected formerly. A healthy and intelligent start for family is important and desirable.

"Today, in our national life the chief problems for most people are not those related to economic well-being but those of uncertainty, anxiety, and fear. Salvation must come through the application of established psychological principles and a better understanding of human relationships. A wisely administered Preparation for Childbirth Program should incluude preparation for the start of family life in order to pay highest dividends.

"The challenge of the future in obstetrical science is based upon the triumphs of the past and the glories of the present and if the American public should become as excited about the problems of human reproduction as it now is about the attack on certain major diseases, benefits would accrue of the profoundest significance.

Given a real public support for research in human reproduction, it is safe to predict that many problems now concerned with pregnancy and labor would be eliminated. The words of Dr. John Rock have significant meaning; 'Yet consider our efforts to learn the nature and life history of the malignant cell, while we neglect the nature and life history of the fertilized egg and how it must be cared for by the mother that both she and her charge will prosper to substantiate the happy family.'

"The real start of family life begins with conception and the more we know about it and its subsequent course the more waste of human life will be eliminated. So, too, the more we can learn about the start of family life and its subsequent course the better we can teach its fundamental principles. Bearing these things in mind, we see that the challenge for the future in obstetrics comes not only to the obstetrician and his co-workers but to all who have a concern in healthy parenthood."

REFERENCES

1. Editorial: *Ladies Home Journal*, April, 1960.
2. Francis, K. D.: (personal communication).
3. Dick Read, G.: (personal communication).
4. Thoms, H.: *Journal of History of Medicine and Allied Sciences.*
5. Thoms, H.: *Our Obstetric Heritage.* Shoestring Press, Hamden, 1960.

INDEX

A

American Association of Obstetricians and Gynecologists, 7
American Association of Nurses Midwifery, 70
American Journal of Obstetrics and Gynecology, 94
American Red Cross, 93
Atlee, H. B., 15, 27, 28, 29, 71, 84, 85

B

Bowley, John, 10
Bradley, J. H., 68
Briefs, 14
Browne, F. J., 4
Bussey, S. C., 3
Buxton, C. L., 11, 71

C

Cadwell, A. B., 46
Catholic Maternity Institute, 71
Columbia-Presbyterian Medical Center, 69, 75
Comparative Study of Reproduction, 6

D

Dalhousie University, 27, 71, 84
Davis, C. D., 7, 18, 23
Deutsche, Helene, 3, 37
Dick Read, Grantly, 4, 6, 7, 19, 24, 77, 78, 90, 94

E

Eastman, N. J., 15, 70, 72, 73, 74, 75
Eliot, Jared, 75
Engelmann, G. J., 6

F

Fairbairn, J. S., 10
Family Centered Maternity Nursing, v, 23, 45

Flower and Fifth Avenue Hospitals, 93
Foord, Alan, 47
Ford Clelland, 6
Frances, K. D., 93
From the Patients' Viewpoint, 14

G

Gesell, Arnold, 47, 64
Goodrich, F. W., v, 5
Grace-New Haven Community Hospital, 48

H

Hayward, Oliver, 79
Heardman, Helen, 4, 6, 25, 30, 90
Hemschemeyer, Hattie, 36
Human Relations in Obstetrical Practice, 12
Hyder, K. H., v, 47

I

Ilg, Frances, 47, 64
International Confederation of Midwives, 70

J

Jackson, E. B., v, vii, 47
Jacobson, Edmund, 4,
Johns Hopkins Hospital, 78
Journal of the History of Medicine, 95
Journal of Obstetrics and Gynaecology of the British Empire, 5

K

Keane, V. R., 14

L

Labor Among Primitive Peoples, 6
Ladies Home Journal, 91
Lancet, The, 12
Lesser, A. J., 70

97